Infodemic in the Era of Post-Truth

With the revolution in information technology, concerns about the proliferation of false, unverified, and misleading information have been growing. As one of the most severe public health crises in modern history, the COVID-19 pandemic has provided a novel context for the "post-truth" research. In a "post-truth" era, people are no longer interested in investigating objective facts, but tend to curl up in echo chambers and resonate with like-minded others. Against this backdrop, this book (1) systematically conceptualises "post-truth" and analyzes its defining characteristics and driving forces, (2) examines the nuanced effects of information sources and news consumption behaviours and strategies on COVID-19 misperceptions and knowledge, (3) explores the role of social media in shaping COVID-19-related misperceptions and knowledge, and (4) highlights the importance of news media literacy in navigating the "post-truth" era.

The book will be essential reading for students and scholars of media and film studies, communication studies and comparative studies. It will also be a useful reference for medical and media professionals such as doctors, nurses and journalists.

Yan Su is an Assistant Professor in the School of Journalism and Communication at Peking University, China. Dr. Su specialises in media effects, emerging communication technologies, health communication, and computational social sciences.

China Perspectives

The *China Perspectives* series focuses on translating and publishing works by leading Chinese scholars, writing about both global topics and China-related themes. It covers Humanities & Social Sciences, Education, Media and Psychology, as well as many interdisciplinary themes.

This is the first time any of these books have been published in English for international readers. The series aims to put forward a Chinese perspective, give insights into cutting-edge academic thinking in China, and inspire researchers globally.

To submit proposals, please contact the Taylor & Francis Publisher for the China Publishing Programme, Lian Sun (Lian.Sun@informa.com)

Titles in media communication currently include:

Cultural Representation and Cultural Studies
Zhou Xian

The "Socialist Transformation" of Memory
Reversing Chinese History through "Pernicious-Vestiges" Media Discourse
Yusi Liu and Ye Ma

Visual Culture in Contemporary China I
Zhou Xian

New Media Users in China I
A Nodes Perspective
Peng Lan

New Media Users in China II
A Mediatization Perspective
Peng Lan

Infodemic in the Era of Post-Truth
Yan Su

For more information, please visit: https://www.routledge.com/China-Perspectives/book-series/CPH

Infodemic in the Era of Post-Truth

Yan Su

Routledge
Taylor & Francis Group

LONDON AND NEW YORK

First published 2024
by Routledge
4 Park Square, Milton Park, Abingdon, Oxon OX14 4RN

and by Routledge
605 Third Avenue, New York, NY 10158

Routledge is an imprint of the Taylor & Francis Group, an informa business

British Library Cataloguing-in-Publication Data
A catalogue record for this book is available from the British Library

Library of Congress Cataloging-in-Publication Data
Names: Su, Yan, 1991- author.
Title: Infodemic in the era of post-truth / Yan Su.
Description: Abingdon, Oxon ; New York, NY : Routledge, 2024. |
Series: China perspectives | Includes bibliographical references and index. | Identifiers: LCCN 2023034055 (print) |
LCCN 2023034056 (ebook) | ISBN 9781032613185 (hardback) |
ISBN 9781032625263 (paperback) | ISBN 9781032625201 (ebook)
Subjects: LCSH: COVID-19 Pandemic, 2020---Social aspects. |
Communication in public health. | Communication--Social aspects. |
Disinformation--Social aspects. | Social media. | COVID-19 (Disease)
Classification: LCC RA644.C67 S82 2024 (print) |
LCC RA644.C67 (ebook) | DDC 610.1/4--dc23/eng/20230828
LC record available at https://lccn.loc.gov/2023034055
LC ebook record available at https://lccn.loc.gov/2023034056

ISBN: 978-1-032-61318-5 (hbk)
ISBN: 978-1-032-62526-3 (pbk)
ISBN: 978-1-032-62520-1 (ebk)

DOI: 10.4324/9781032625201

Typeset in Times New Roman
by SPi Technologies India Pvt Ltd (Straive)

Contents

Introduction and Background

Upon being named as the 2016's word of the year, the "post-truth" phenomenon has started to gain extensive scholarly attention. In a "post-truth" era, people no longer perceive objective facts as relevant or important, instead, they are prone to curl up in echo chambers, seeking for resonance among like-minded others. The arrival of the "post-truth" era was mainly driven by the technological empowerment, the deepening postmodernism, and the consistent decline in the public's confidence in governments and the scientific community.

The postmodernist culture has fueled the trend of individualism and decentralization, further leading to challenges to the monopolistic elite discourse system. The appeal to the openness to representational systems and the rebellion against elitism has resulted in the decline of authoritative narratives, while individual, even populist, narratives have become acceptable alternative interpretations of objective existence. The deepening of the postmodernity has paved a way for the emergence of misinformation. The revolution of information technologies has further allowed for the uncurbed circulation of false, unverified, and misleading information. However, the "post-truth" state does not merely entail the existence of falsehoods, it also denotes the fact that people start to concentrate less on facts and more on emotional appeals as they navigate the environment in which a variety of information, misinformation, and conspiracy theories are intertwined.

As one of the most severe public health crises in modern history, the COVID-19 pandemic has provided a novel context for the "post-truth" research. Amidst the pandemic, the director-general Tedros Adhanom Ghebreyesus of the World Health Organization indicated that "We're not just fighting a pandemic; we're fighting an infodemic." An "infodemic" describes the state that verified and unverified health information interweaved, which makes it difficult for people to find reliable sources and guidance. The extant literature on misinformation and the "post-truth" phenomenon, notwithstanding growing rapidly, has not yet lent sufficient credence to their antecedents, nor has it provided constructive and systematic recommendations to alleviate these phenomena.

Against this backdrop, this book has the following research purposes. First and foremost, this book systematically conceptualizes the "post-truth" era,

DOI: 10.4324/9781032625201-1

identifying its characteristics, and more importantly, analyzing its driving forces. The book highlights that the joint force of the technological empowerment, the deepening of postmodernism, and the consistent decline in the public trust in political institutions and authorities has fuelled and accelerated the arrival of the "post-truth" era.

Second, using survey data, this book empirically examines the nuanced conditional indirect effects of information source utilizations and news exposure styles on misperceptions and factual knowledge about the COVID-19 pandemic. Specifically, this book investigates the influence of partisan media use on people's misperceptions through affecting their risk perceptions about the pandemic and avoidance behaviors such as message derogation. It also probes whether these impacts are contingent upon people's political ideology, the extent to which they trust medical experts, their need for cognition, perceived media locus of control, and their discussion network homogeneity. Apart from the effect of information sources (i.e., partisan media), this book further explores whether incidental exposure to traditional mass media and ambient news awareness could affect people's misperceptions and factual knowledge with respect to the pandemic. These attempts are committed to exploring the very antecedents of the formation of the COVID-19-related misperceptions and the factual knowledge about the COVID-19.

Third, as social media platforms have been deemed as a fertile breeding ground for misinformation to circulate, this book takes a step further and empirically probes the role of social media news exposure, both proactively and incidentally, in shaping people's misperceptions and factual knowledge of the COVID-19 pandemic. Considering that echo chambers and filter bubbles prevailed in social media spheres, preventing people from encountering social corrections and diversified viewpoints, this book takes a step further and explores whether the impacts of social media use on COVID-19 misperceptions and knowledge are contingent upon people's discussion network heterogeneity.

Fourth, upon unravelling the various communication factors that might contribute to this "post-truth" phenomenon, this book empirically investigates the role of news media literacy. This book argues that due to the irreversibility of the three driving forces, namely, the technological empowerment, the deepening postmodernism, and the consistent decline in public trust in authorities, that any idea that the "post-truth" state will only persist briefly is wrong. On the contrary, the current cognitive dilemma caused by the "post-truth" phenomenon is more likely an inevitable part of the process of knowledge democratization. As such, through empirical analyses, this book puts forth that the silver lining lies at people's good news media literacy and critical thinking abilities. In essence, this analysis is committed to rendering constructive suggestions for institutions and individuals to prevent the adverse consequences of the "infodemic" while navigating this "post-truth" era.

In the remainder of this book, each chapter is committed to achieving each of the above-mentioned research purposes. That is, Chapter 1 defines the concept of the "post-truth," analyzes its characteristics, and identifies its driving forces. Chapter 2 builds a series of regression models based on two survey samples from the United States and China, respectively, to explore the effects of information source utilization and news exposure methods. Chapter 3 continues the quantitative analysis of the survey samples from the two countries, discussing the impact of social media use. Chapter 4 discusses the role of news media literacy through quantitative survey data analysis. Chapter 5 is a summary of the main points of the previous chapters.

It bears mentioning that the analyses of samples in two countries, the U.S. and China, is much warranted due to the following factors. First, both countries were at the epicentre of public opinions revolving around the COVID-19 pandemic. Moreover, both countries have large markets of conspiracy theories. Last but not least, the two countries have distinct media landscape and culture, which helps reveal the nuances of media effects across different political and cultural settings, providing insights into different theoretical and practical implications.

1   Conceptualizing the "Post-truth"

After the Oxford Dictionaries named "post-truth" 2016's word of the year, the phenomenon swiftly gained widespread public attention around the world. The alleged "post-truth" does not merely encompass fake news, lies, fabrications, or deceits, but also involves the public's reactions to them. Compared with facts and scientific evidence of controversial issues, the public's emotional resonance has become increasingly important. In other words, in a "post-truth" era, people are no longer interested in exploring objective facts, instead, they are more prone to seek for emotional appeals and echoes among like-minded others. The emerging communication technology and its rich technological affordances have endowed its users with unique opportunities to practice consumptive news feeds curation and selective exposure to the greatest extent (Majchrzak et al., 2013; Messing & Westwood, 2014). Technology users can curate their consumptive feeds to avoid discordance and conflict, thereby avoiding the cognitive dissonance (Metzger et al., 2020) and continuously expanding their homogeneous networks. In this case, affective polarization is greatly intensified, leading to multiple adverse societal ramifications.

In the compound word "post-truth", the subcomponent term "post" does not denote the time after a particular event as in the similar words "post-war" or "post-operative care;" Instead, the "post" in the "post-truth" refers to a state in which the specified concept is no longer relevant or important. Therefore, the term "post-truth" should be understood as the state where truths are not deemed important anymore. Akin to the meaning of the "post-truth," the "post-racial" also refers to the state in which racial relations are no longer considered relevant.

The arrival of the "post-truth" era and the emergence of the "post-truth politics" have undoubtedly posed a solemn challenge to a healthy democracy (Rose, 2017; Suiter, 2016). Admittedly, before Trump's unexpected victory in 2016, the political advertizements and debates were already filled with all kinds of misinformation and lies. However, not akin to those previous politicians, Trump stood out by his outspokenly disdainful attitude towards truths and facts. Trump has shown his disdain so verbally and explicitly as if he had discovered that the democratic myth that made everyone tremble was just a counterfeit. For the first time, the democratic world has encountered an outspoken

DOI: 10.4324/9781032625201-2

"post-truth politician" who has never bothered utilizing any politicians' filters in any public occasions. Trump, however, aptly identified that American political rhetoric has already become hollow, full of platitudes and hypocrisy that have nothing to do with truths. However, the ways in which Trump navigates politics is by creating and spreading more lies, using one rumor after another to whitewash himself and justify his rule.

Many commentators lamented that the scale of Trump's mendacity was unprecedented in the history of the U.S. politics. According to the tally of *The Washington Post*, Trump created and disseminated 21 lies per day during his presidency. However, his supporters seemed to have remained steadfast and loyal. The disastrous consequences of the post-truth politics are by no means merely confined to the increase in after-dinner conversations, the Capitol attack in 2021, for instance, was a more direct blow to the existing political institutions and even the entire democratic process. Although post-truth politics has facilitated the decentralization and the alleged democratization of expression, the calamitous consequences of populism will only challenge or even disintegrate a good democratic system, forming a vicious circle. Indeed, we have also seen clearly in the past few years that although this kind of "post-truth politics" brings a moment of joy, it makes the democratic politics fall into the dark abyss.

In addition, the various misinformation, disinformation, malinformation, fake news, and conspiracy theories relevant to the COVID-19 pandemic and the irreparable social losses these theories have caused became a profound lesson for the entire mankind. Because of these misinformation and conspiracy theories, many people unfortunately missed the best time and the most effective measures to prevent the virus. It is no exaggeration to say that too many lives have been lost due to misinformation. Therefore, upon recalling such painful experiences, we urgently need to reach the consensus that the truth is good. Truths can sometimes make people uncomfortable, and some truths are far less fascinating than most of the conspiracy theories, but only with rational, fact-based solutions can we expect a democratic society to truly thrive.

In this Chapter, I argue that the very antecedents, or driving forces, of the post-truth phenomenon can be divided into three categories, namely, the technological empowerment, the deepening of postmodernism, and the consistent decline in public trust in government.

The first driving force, the technological empowerment, mainly entails the novel opportunities brought about to the public by the emerging communication technologies such as social media. Apart from the fact that authoritative discourse is no longer paid attention to, and that scientists are not taken seriously anymore, the rise and ubiquity of emerging communication technologies also affected people's perceptions of the overall information environment, resulting in fundamental changes in news consumption habits, which in turn solidifies people's dependence on the algorithmic mechanisms and their social networks. In fact, this leaves a huge space for platform manipulation and the formation of algorithmic Leviathans (Creel & Hellman, 2022; König, 2020).

The instinct to avoid cognitive dissonance has always existed (Festinger, 1957), even in offline settings, people strive to avoid potential confrontations through switching topics when discordance or conflicting ideas are detected, but due to the lack of technological empowerment, the initiative of avoiding cognitive dissonance and selectively exposing oneself only to certain like-minded contents, has not been fully activated. Social media have offered this possibility through abundant technological affordances. Specifically, I argue that the driving force of technological empowerment is further reflected in two specific aspects, namely, the algorithms and the popularity of weak ties.

The first aspect in which the technological empowerment reflects is the popularization of algorithm news. The growth of digital media has severely undermined and eroded the traditional gatekeeper role that journalists played, giving birth to a new form of gatekeeping based on artificial intelligence, centered around algorithmic news selection and editing (DeVito, 2017; Gil de Zúñiga et al., 2022). Thorson and Wells (2016) have identified five sets of curating actors in today's social media news exposure, namely, "journalists, strategic communicators, individual media users (personal curators), social contacts, and algorithmic filters" (p. 314). Algorithm curation refers to the alleged invisible decisions that algorithmis make regarding what content should be showcased to a user (Braun & Gillespie, 2011; Thorson & Wells, 2016), which complicates the other four types of curators.

As a part of the online communication infrastructure, algorithm curation is deemed a culprit for the formation of filter bubbles, an algorithmic bias skewing and confining the scope of news and information an individual Internet user would see on their feeds (Pariser, 2011; Slechten et al., 2022). More specifically, the algorithms curate feeds and facilitate the creation of filter bubbles through two major approaches, namely, the user-based curation and the content-based curation. First, through constantly recommending other users with homogeneous characteristics to one user, the algorithms invisibly facilitate the connections among users with similar features and promote the development of online homophily. If things move on like this, people will inevitably encounter more users that the algorithms deemed similar to them in the online spheres while being more alienated from heterogeneous users and having less chances to encounter differences (Brundidge, 2010). Second, through tracking and documenting a user's browsing records, the algorithm recommend information homogeneous to what the user consumed in the past or what it deems favourable to the user, strengthening their path dependency on consuming certain type of contents.

Either way, algorithms would solidify and crystallize the online echo chambers, encouraging people to expose to like-minded viewpoints more frequently, and thus lose the opportunity to expose to heterogeneous opinions. However, political discussion is deemed the soul of a deliberative democracy, while only heterogeneous discussions could facilitate the free flow of pluralistic and diversified information (Cinelli et al., 2021; Haim et al., 2018). The algorithmic curation, as an increasingly irreplaceable part of the online communication infrastructure, allows the resonance of homogeneous opinions that intensifies affective and ideological polarization, hastening the arrival of the "post-truth" era. An experiment did illustrate that the emotional states of emerging communication technology users can be significantly affected by algorithmic selection and curation (Kramer et al., 2014). Simultaneously, a solemn concern with respect to the deepening of the gap between the information rich and the information poor has also risen, in that information and knowledge will be accumulated exponentially for people who already of a higher socioeconomic status and of more abundant social capitals (Thorson & Wells, 2016).

The second aspect of technological driving force is reflected in the popularity of weak ties on social media platforms. Granovetter (1973) used to have a rosy imagination of weak ties, but even though the strengths of weak ties are confirmed in the context of job hunting, weak ties in the online spheres do not always have positive and constructive societal ramifications. For instance, scholars have raised concerns about the alleged networked individualism brought about by weak ties (Foth & Hearn, 2007; Wellman, 2002; Wellman et al., 2003). Specifically, people's growing reluctance to engage in civic activities has resulted in a severe decline in social cohesion, a breakdown in trust between individuals, widespread loneliness, and reduced ability for people to act collectively in solidarity. These will certainly deepen the drawbacks and challenges of the "post-truth" era.

For instance, the "online slacktivism" will be fostered, and people will hold firmly that the mere utilization of technological affordances for emotional and attitudinal expressions would be sufficient to solve all problems (Kwak et al., 2018; Lane & Dal Cin, 2018). Over time, people will become increasingly unwilling to participate in civic affairs and fulfill their civic responsibilities. Online slacktivism precisely entails the belief that clicking "likes" or sharing posts could suffice most of the demands of social movements. Social media users typically spend a lot of time seeking virtual gratification, which undermines and weakens the incentive and motivation to participate in offline politics in that they would only like to participate when they are sure that the movement requires no real sacrifice. In addition, as opinion expression becomes more convenient in social media platforms, the average value of each opinion will be weakened, which makes it more difficult for opinions to create a real impact. Hence, technologically empowered expressions are likely not to fundamentally change any status quos, but to make the existing social order more efficient and solidified.

In addition to technological empowerment, the second driving force pertains to the deepening of postmodernism. Modernism holds that texts, representations, and symbols are closed systems, and any concept can only have a unique, accurate, and authoritative definition. However, postmodernism does the opposite, arguing that texts, representations, and symbols are open systems, and there should be an infinite number of ways of interpretations of any concept (Cetina, 1994; Hassan, 1985; Soffer, 2009). As Bauman (1988) suggested, postmodernity denotes a trend in aestheticism keyed to "increased individualism," multiple choices, self-enrichment, and self-enlargement (Cetina, 1994, p. 1). In other words, postmodern culture emphasizes interpretive flexibility, encouraging individuals to define, interpret, and explicate concepts regardless of any authoritative or monopolistic discourses (Cetina, 1994; Habermas, 1983). From a philosophical point of view, postmodernists often harbor a skeptical attitude toward logical concepts and structural interpretations. This attitude typically results in a serious lack of desire for ideas, materials, and external sensations, because from the postmodernists' perspective, their thinking has no way to rely on. In other words, postmodernists neither affirm historical experience nor believe in the authenticity of any constructed facts and their meanings.

Gadamer (1975) argued that human's understanding of all existence is essentially based on language as a universal medium, and language is also the structural factor of all interpretations. Hence, the world we perceive is constructed by language, and therefore, our mastery of language is where the boundaries of our understanding lie. However, one of the appeals of postmodernism is to go beyond the solidified framework of the understanding composed of the elements such as rationality, integrity, central duality, and structuralism. Therefore, postmodernists began to seek innovations in the construction of new languages. With the deepening of the postmodern culture, we have even witnessed a potential transformation in journalism industry, that is, the turn from professional journalism toward dialectic journalism. Such transformation undoubtedly poses a glaringly severe challenge toward the occupational ideology, professional culture, and sedimentation of routines of the traditional journalism industry (Deuze & Witschge, 2018).

Then, how has it to do with the characteristics of the "post-truth" era? As postmodernist notions take hold, the alleged facts could simply be seen as different versions of the narrative; lies can be argued to be another point of view or opinions because everything is relative, and everyone are endowed the right to define their own truth and construct their own reality. It is undeniable that postmodernism deems itself to be emancipatory and freeing people from the monopoly and oppression of authoritative narratives and discourses. However, media populism also comes with it (Krämer, 2014). If facts and reality become malleable, governments can legitimize wars of aggression merely based on misinformation and malinformation they themselves created. The Bush administration could deftly defend its invasion to Iraq, and the Trump administration can also legitimize all its COVID-19 policies simply based on the conspiracy theories that the then-President had fabricated, endorsed, or facilitated (Borah et al., 2022; Evanega et al., 2020). More worryingly, through declaring that all knowledge is of an oppressive nature, postmodernism effectively strips away the grounded arguments against power. Instead, it holds that rationality and intellectualism are forms of domination, and that people must seek revolutionary liberation through their emotions. Therefore, the preference of emotions to fact-based arguments thus gains legitimacy.

Amid the COVID-19 pandemic, people have shown unprecedented distrust of public health experts and scientists yet become more prone to trust politicians who share their ideology. A large number of American citizens seemed to turn a blind eye to the scientific evidence presented by the scientific community but are keen to express, on various social media platforms, their endorsement of certain conspiracy theories such as those related to the 5G networks, Bill Gates, Agenda 21, and QAnon (Himelboim et al., 2023). These phenomena are vivid manifestations of postmodernism's empowerment of individualism, self-enrichment, and self-enlargement. There is little doubt that these post-modernism-based Internet chaos have intensified the long-standing vaccination hesitancy among the U.S. citizens (Kreps et al., 2021), hindering people from enacting recommended preventive measures such as vaccination, mask wearing, and social distancing.

Conspiracy theories themselves are of a strong deconstructive nature. As part of the postmodern counter-attack process against the structuralism, some specific strategies of deconstructionism have a guiding significance for weaving conspiracy theories and reinterpreting complex issues. In particular, when the amount of information is asymmetric, and the right to reveal and interpret the truth is in the hands of individual authorities, postmodernists can easily use conspiracy theories to deconstruct authoritative narratives that they do not buy, so as to re-attribute and resituate the inexplicably complex phenomenon. The famous conspiracy theories related to the 9/11 and moon landing are exactly reflections of this logical process. In sum, at a time when postmodernist culture has become deeply ingrained, people have already formed a habitual rebellion against authoritative narratives and definitions. Especially when these explanations and definitions fail to satisfy the public, the public would choose to believe in conspiracy theories that seem to have more explanatory power and are more self-justifying, and act under the guidance of the conspiracy theories.

The third driving force of the arrival of the "post-truth" era, apart from the technological empowerment and the deepening of the postmodernism, involves the long-standing public disaffection with government. If we only focus on the technology's role in activating individuals' initiatives in consumptive news feeds curation and empowering their practices of selective exposure without paying attention to the public's long-term dissatisfaction with the political institutions, the public policies, the political climate, or the economic status, we would not only fall into the narrow perspective of the technological determinism, but also not be able to make sense of how misinformation circulates so rampantly. In fact, technology itself only provides a channel for its users to express dissatis-faction. Even social media, which is full of multimodal information and offers multiple technological affordances such as liking, commenting, and retweeting, still only lends a channel for their users to express attitudes and opinions. What we should pay more attention to is the fact that the public's disaffection with political institutions and figures has been building up for a long time.

Recent Pew polls showed a consistent decline in public trust in government among the U.S. citizens for over sixty years (e.g., Pew Research Centre, 2022). Admittedly, the erosion of public trust in government began in the 1960s, when the escalation of the Vietnam War and the subsequent Watergate scandal fueled the tendency. It slightly recovered in the mid-1980s notwithstanding, the public trust in government swiftly declined again at the very beginning of the 21st Century. Thereafter, the public trust in government has never surpassed 30%. With Trump's unexpected victory in 2016, people have witnessed a rapid intensification and deterioration of the affective polarization among the U.S. citizens.

When it comes to the public confidence in the scientific community, a Pew poll released in 2022 exhibited that trust in medical scientists, which once appeared to be buoyed by their key role in responding to the COVID-19 pandemic, was now below the pre-pandemic level. Specifically, tallies in November 2020 showed that 40% of the surveyed U.S. citizens indicated that they have a great deal of confidence in medical experts that they would act in the best interest of the general public, whereas the statistics has dropped to 29% in 2022 (Pew Research Centre, 2022). This data undoubtedly sounded an alarm for us.

Even without the sudden outbreak of the COVID-19 pandemic, people from both extremes of the ideological spectrum have already been constantly struggling over issues such as the climate change, tax policies, immigration policies, and infrastructure policies. The COVID-19 pandemic and its lingering impact on the entire country have just rendered a new theme for new rounds of political rants, struggles, and attacks, accelerating the highlighting of structural difficulties of the "post-truth" era. Even more so, the COVID-19 pandemic was perhaps the final straw that breaks the camel's back; people have been burdened with a series of issues, while the outbreak of the pandemic at a time when people are on the brink of being overwhelmed just offered an opportunity for them to express their long-term disaffection fully and freely. It is clear that the attribute agendas under the first-level issue agenda (i.e., the virus per se), were in fact highly related to many political debate topics that have existed for long. For instance, the unfounded conspiracy theory regarding the lab leak in Wuhan is nothing more than another manifestation of the long-standing hatred and fear of the Communist China; and the theory that Bill Gates was committed to profiting from vaccination may also be a representation of the public's long-standing disgust towards the subterfuge of capitalists and politicians. Emerging communication technologies are nothing more than endowing people with the conditionalities, under which they can express their emotions and attitudes using multimodal information and rich affordances. Hence, the unique landscape of this unprecedented "infodemic" has taken shape right under our noses.

In sum, the defining characteristics of the "post-truth" era are not shaped by a single factor but are driven by the combined force of the technological empowerment, the deepening of postmodernism, and the long-standing public disaffection with the authorities. It is precisely because of the irreversibility of these three driving forces that any idea that the "post-truth" state will only persist briefly is undoubtedly wrong. On the contrary, it would be in our real interest to view the current cognitive dilemma caused by the "post-truth" state as an inevitable part of the painful process of information democratization. Regardless of the fact that we may not be able to return to the era before the "post-truth" era, as the "post-truth" phenomenon has indiscriminately destroyed all kinds of institutions and systems, including good ones, we cannot sit idly by, but we need to consider seriously the constructive approaches through which we can develop critical thinking and skills, so as to better navigate and live healthily in this "post truth" era.

References

Bauman, Z. (1988). Is there a postmodern sociology? *Theory, Culture & Society*, 5(2–3), 217–237.

Borah, P., Austin, E., & Su, Y. (2022). Injecting disinfectants to kill the virus: Media literacy, information gathering sources, and the moderating role of political ideology on misperceptions about COVID-19. *Mass Communication & Society*, 1–27.

Braun, J., & Gillespie, T. (2011). Hosting the public discourse, hosting the public: When online news and social media converge. *Journalism Practice*, 5(4), 383–398.

Brundidge, J. (2010). Encountering "difference" in the contemporary public sphere: The contribution of the Internet to the heterogeneity of political discussion networks. *Journal of Communication*, 60(4), 680–700.

Cetina, K. K. (1994). Primitive classification and postmodernity: Towards a sociological notion of fiction. *Theory, Culture & Society*, 11(3), 1–22.

Cinelli, M., De Francisci Morales, G., Galeazzi, A., Quattrociocchi, W., & Starnini, M. (2021). The echo chamber effect on social media. *Proceedings of the National Academy of Sciences*, 118(9), e2023301118.

Creel, K., & Hellman, D. (2022). The algorithmic Leviathan: Arbitrariness, fairness, and opportunity in algorithmic decision-making systems. *Canadian Journal of Philosophy*, 52(1), 26–43.

Deuze, M., & Witschge, T. (2018). Beyond journalism: Theorizing the transformation of journalism. *Journalism*, 19(2), 165–181.

DeVito, M. A. (2017). From editors to algorithms: A values-based approach to understanding story selection in the Facebook news feed. *Digital Journalism*, 5(6), 753–773.

Evanega, S., Lynas, M., Adams, J., Smolenyak, K., & Insights, C. G. (2020). Coronavirus misinformation: Quantifying sources and themes in the COVID-19 'infodemic'. *JMIR Preprints*, 19(10), 2020.

Festinger, L. (1957). *A theory of cognitive dissonance*. Evanstone, IL: Row, Peterson.

Foth, M., & Hearn, G. (2007). Networked individualism of urban residents: Discovering the communicative ecology in inner-city apartment buildings. *Information, Communication & Society*, 10(5), 749–772.

Gadamer, H. (1975). *Truth and Method*. London: Sheed and Ward

Gil de Zúñiga, H., Cheng, Z., & González-González, P. (2022). Effects of the News Finds Me perception on algorithmic news attitudes and social media political homophily. *Journal of Communication*, 72(5), 578–591.

Granovetter, M. S. (1973). The strength of weak ties. *American Journal of Sociology*, 78(6), 1360–1380.

Habermas, J. (1983) *Theory of Communicative Action*. Boston: Beacon.

Haim, M., Graefe, A., & Brosius, H. B. (2018). Burst of the filter bubble? Effects of personalization on the diversity of Google News. *Digital Journalism*, 6(3), 330–343.

Hassan, I. (1985). The culture of postmodernism. *Theory, Culture & Society*, 2(3), 119–131.

Himelboim, I., Borah, P., Lee, D. K. L., Lee, J., Su, Y., Vishnevskaya, A., & Xiao, X. (2023). What do 5G networks, Bill Gates, Agenda 21, and QAnon have in common? Sources, distribution, and characteristics. *New Media & Society*, 1–21.

König, P. D. (2020). Dissecting the algorithmic leviathan: On the socio-political anatomy of algorithmic governance. *Philosophy & Technology*, *33*(3), 467–485.

Kramer, A. D. I., Guillory, J. E., & Hancock, J. T. (2014). Experimental evidence of massive-scale emotional contagion through social networks. *Proceedings of the National Academy of Sciences*, *111*(24), 8788–8790.

Krämer, B. (2014). Media populism: A conceptual clarification and some theses on its effects. *Communication Theory*, *24*(1), 42–60.

Kreps, S. E., Goldfarb, J. L., Brownstein, J. S., & Kriner, D. L. (2021). The relationship between US adults' misconceptions about COVID-19 vaccines and vaccination preferences. *Vaccines*, *9*(8), 901.

Kwak, N., Lane, D. S., Weeks, B. E., Kim, D. H., Lee, S. S., & Bachleda, S. (2018). Perceptions of social media for politics: Testing the slacktivism hypothesis. *Human Communication Research*, *44*(2), 197–221.

Lane, D. S., & Dal Cin, S. (2018). Sharing beyond Slacktivism: The effect of socially observable prosocial media sharing on subsequent offline helping behavior. *Information, Communication & Society*, *21*(11), 1523–1540.

Majchrzak, A., Faraj, S., Kane, G. C., & Azad, B. (2013). The contradictory influence of social media affordances on online communal knowledge sharing. *Journal of Computer-Mediated Communication*, *19*(1), 38–55.

Messing, S., & Westwood, S. J. (2014). Selective exposure in the age of social media: Endorsements trump partisan source affiliation when selecting news online. *Communication Research*, *41*(8), 1042–1063.

Metzger, M. J., Hartsell, E. H., & Flanagin, A. J. (2020). Cognitive dissonance or credibility? A comparison of two theoretical explanations for selective exposure to partisan news. *Communication Research*, *47*(1), 3–28.

Pariser, E. (2011). *The filter bubble: What the internet is hiding from you*. New York, NY: Penguin Press

Pew Research Centre. (2022). Public Trust in Government: 1958–2022. https://www. pewresearch.org/politics/2022/06/06/public-trust-in-government-1958-2022/

Rose, J. (2017). Brexit, Trump, and post-truth politics. *Public Integrity*, *19*(6), 555–558.

Slechten, L., Courtois, C., Coenen, L., & Zaman, B. (2022). Adapting the selective exposure perspective to algorithmically governed platforms: The case of Google Search. *Communication Research*, *49*(8), 1039–1065.

Soffer, O. (2009). The competing ideals of objectivity and dialogue in American journalism. *Journalism*, *10*(4), 473–491.

Suiter, J. (2016). Post-truth politics. *Political insight*, *7*(3), 25–27.

Thorson, K., & Wells, C. (2016). Curated flows: A framework for mapping media exposure in the digital age. *Communication Theory*, *26*(3), 309–328

Wellman, B., Quan-Haase, A., Boase, J., Chen, W., Hampton, K., Díaz, I., & Miyata, K. (2003). The social affordances of the Internet for networked individualism. *Journal of Computer-Mediated Communication*, *8*(3), JCMC834.

Wellman, B. (2002, July). Little boxes, glocalization, and networked individualism. In *Digital cities II: Computational and sociological approaches: Second Kyoto workshop on digital cities Kyoto, Japan, October 18–20, 2001 Revised Papers* (pp. 10–25). Berlin, Heidelberg: Springer Berlin Heidelberg.

2 Information Sources and News Consumption Habitus

This chapter continues the discussion of the "post-truth era," whilst it focuses more on the antecedents of it. In specific, this chapter examines the nuanced media effects on the formation of misperceptions in the context of the COVID-19 pandemic. Communication variables can be divided by whether the media is elite-gatekept (legacy media vs. social media), partisanships of the media (conservative media vs. liberal media), and the consumption patterns among news consumers (incidental news exposure vs. proactive news seeking). This chapter seeks to establish an account as to what type(s) of information source and news consumption behavior(s) are associated with higher extents of misperceptions, taking into consideration the exogenous variables such as individuals' demographics and other psychological factors. The analysis and argument of this chapter will be based on survey samples from the U.S. and China. In a nutshell, this chapter is committed to heeding the call to provide empirical evidence for the causes and antecedents of misperceptions, from the theoretical perspective of media effects.

2.1 Partisan Media Use and COVID-19 Misperceptions

2.1.1 COVID-19 Misinformation and Misperceptions

Misinformation is conceptualized as false or inaccurate information, which has ballooned exponentially in various media outlets. Research on misinformation has proliferated in recent years, particularly after Brexit and Trump's unexpected win in the 2016 U.S. Presidential Election. Researchers have thus devoted more efforts in studying misinformation in the realm of politics. Studies in this vein include both antecedents and consequences of misinformation, as well as the countermeasures of political misinformation (e.g., Li, 2020; Schaffner & Luks, 2018). With the emergence of the COVID-19 pandemic, health-related misinformation and conspiracy theories have been rampantly circulating through various channel outlets, generating a new agenda of research. For instance, scholars have examined the structure and organization of beliefs in pandemic conspiracy theories and misinformation (Enders et al., 2020) and the magnitude of misinformation that is being spread on Twitter regarding the

DOI: 10.4324/9781032625201-3

COVID-19 pandemic (Kouzy et al., 2020). Himelboim and associates (2023) investigated the information sources, typology, and building blocks of the major conspiracy theories on Twitter during the COVID-19 pandemic.

One of the severe consequences of being misinformed is the formation of misperception. Misperception is defined as "cases in which people's beliefs about factual matters are not supported by clear evidence and expert opinion" (Nyhan & Reifler, 2010, p. 305). The proliferation of misinformation and persistent misperceptions could cause a wide range of detrimental consequences that may inflict harm on the intellectual well-being of society. A panoply of studies has documented the destructive influences of misinformation and misperception such as causing public health crises, eroding trust in experts and authoritative and scientific institutions, intensifying discrimination and xenophobia, and even stirring up social chaos and turmoil (Enders et al., 2020; Lee et al., 2023; Malik et al., 2023; Silvia Chou et al., 2020; Southwell et al., 2019; Stubenvoll et al., 2021).

Oftentimes, misinformation thrives on controversial issues and debates, particularly in the realms of health and science (Benegal & Scruggs, 2018; Farrell et al., 2019; West & Bergstrom, 2021). A large proportion of research has been dedicated to the investigation of the predictors and consequences of misperceptions with regard to the environmental issues such as climate change (Ballew et al., 2020; Chinn & Pasek, 2021; Kerr & Wilson, 2018; Lata & Nunn, 2012; Moxnes & Saysel, 2009; Nyhan, 2020, 2021). In the realm of health communication, plenty of studies have also examined the role of misinformation in shaping people's certain behavioral intentions such as vaccine hesitancy, a common psychological tendency that has already generated a large variety of conspiracy theories. Despite the fact that the vaccination is one of the most cost-effective public health interventions and the vast amount of evidence of the validity and functionality of vaccines rendered by the extent research, vaccine hesitancy has still been growing significantly among U.S. citizens, triggering the inability of epidemic containment and resulting in prominence and prevalence of anti-intellectualism as well as decreased trust of experts (Chou & Budenz, 2020; Goldenberg, 2016). The contributing factors of vaccine hesitancy are manifold, and misinformation is among these factors (Hornsey et al., 2020). Besides, individuals' limited science literacy, low risk perceptions of health crises, broken trust in the scientific community, decreased perceived expectancies of vaccines, and reduced perceived susceptibility are all significant contributing factors of vaccine hesitancy (Biasio, 2017; Krieger & Sarge, 2013; Myrick, 2017; Nan et al., 2015; Smith et al., 2017; Wilson et al., 2020).

Following the outbreak of the COVID-19, fabricated stories, misinformation, disinformation, mal-information, fake news, and conspiracy theories have occupied various mass media outlets and social media platforms, causing much confusion among the public and delaying public health actions (Enders et al., 2020). For instance, people erroneously believe that the origin of the coronavirus was associated with the 5G mobile network or the Wuhan Institute of Virology (Ahmed et al., 2020; Cuan-Baltazar et al., 2020); some are extremely convinced that Bill Gates and the related conglomerates were using the COVID-19 pandemic for their depopulation purposes or to implant tracking devices in humans with COVID-19 vaccination (Shahsavari et al., 2020); many others even blatantly defy preventive guidelines and refuse to take precautionary measurements such as wearing masks and social distancing because they deemed the pandemic a total hoax (e.g., Hornik et al., 2021). Scholars warned that conspiracy beliefs regarding COVID-19 could lead to lower compliance with social distancing measures (Bridgman et al., 2020), reluctance to abide by the mask mandate (Morris, 2021), and greater vaccine hesitancy (Lazarus et al., 2022), which is consistent with the general literature on vaccines and risk perception (Detoc et al., 2020; Karafillakis & Larson, 2017). According to Lazarus and associates (2022), individuals with heavy misperceptions may "reflect a respondent's lower trust in the science behind vaccine research and production" (p. 7), aligning a series of existing literature in the same vein of research (e.g., Bicchieri et al., 2021; Cadeddu et al., 2020; May, 2020; Palamenghi et al., 2020; Veit et al., 2021). Taken together, widespread misinformation and subsequent misperceptions in the domain of health may deter and undermine the public health and environmental protection efforts and actions.

2.1.2 *Partisan Media in the United States*

Plenty of research has lent sufficient credence with respect to the effects of news media on individuals' perceptions of reality. Consuming news from mass media is a key predictor of social learning, knowledge acquisition, and perception formation, which further influences people's attitudes and even behaviors. A series of classic theories in communication research, such as the agenda-setting theory, the social cognitive theory, the differential gains model, and the communication mediation model precisely describe the above mechanism, providing rich empirical evidence in the past few decades (Eveland Jr., 2001; McCombs & Shaw, 1972; Scheufele, 2002; Shah et al., 2017).

That being said, the above-mentioned outcomes of media use do not always accumulate uniformly in that people's ideological stances and pre-existing values and beliefs could affect the ways in which they grasp the information and make sense of the news and information they were exposed to (Garrett et al., 2019; Su et al., 2022). These pre-existing ideologies could lead people to selectively expose to certain contents that are congruent with their beliefs in order to avoid cognitive dissonance (Sears & Freedman, 1967). This phenomenon is also closely tied to motivated reasoning. To be specific, motivated reasoning describes the situation that individuals usually on a biased set of cognitive processes during reasoning, according to specific goals (Bolsen et al., 2014; Kunda, 1990). Two essential goals within motivated reasoning are accuracy and directional goals (Kunda, 1990). Individuals are inclined to spend more cognitive efforts on issue-related reasoning and elaborate on relevant information when they were driven by accuracy goals while striving for the desired conclusion that conforms to their predispositions when driven by directional goals (Bayes & Druckman, 2021; Druckman & McGrath, 2019). Although motivated reasoning comprises both directional and accuracy goals, researchers generally use the term to refer to directional goals and directional reasoning (Bayes & Druckman, 2021). Motivated reasoning has been widely employed to explain the divergent or polarized opinion landscape in the contexts of environmental (Bayes & Druckman, 2021; Hart & Nisbet, 2012) and health issues (Freiling et al., 2023). Since the concept of motivated reasoning pertains to people's intentions to reach particular conclusions congruent with pre-existing beliefs (e.g., political party identification) (Bolsen et al., 2014), it is closely related to the classical communication mediation model wherein the moderator are individual's cognitive dispositions and motivational characteristics (McLeod et al., 1994). As a part of the initial orientation, motivated reasoning affects not only how audiences interpret messages but also how they consume news (Cho et al., 2009). For instance, in order to maintain a sense of political identification and relieve cognitive stress, individuals are likely to turn to corresponding partisan media for attitude-consistent information (Knobloch-Westerwick & Meng, 2009; Su et al., 2022). Moreover, motivated reasoning propels people to seek information that fits existing beliefs and dismiss counter-belief information simultaneously, regardless of the accuracy of the certain belief (Bolsen et al., 2014). Partisan media serve as an ideal space to encounter such belief-consistent messages, especially for contentious and politicized issues (Chung & Jones-Jang, 2022).

In the United States, partisan media have long been criticized for creating chaos and fueling confusion regarding significant societal issues, as well as contributing to controversies and affective and ideological polarization among citizens (e.g., Levendusky, 2013; Stroud, 2010). Partisan media are "outlets that cover news and politics in a way that favors one political party or ideology over others, and offer opinionated coverage (Weeks et al., 2021, p. 3), and these media outlets often promote partisan viewpoints through biased descriptions in their stories either explicitly or implicitly (Levendusky, 2013). For instance, opinion content included in Fox News and MSNBC demonstrate a distinct bias toward Republican and Democrat perspectives, respectively (Su et al., 2022). In specific, Fox News exhibited a congruently pro-Republican slant (Iyengar & Hahn, 2009), hence, it is deemed the right-wing blogosphere (Skocpol & Williamson, 2016; Su et al., 2022). A plethora of studies has operationalized right-wing media utilization as individuals' frequencies with which they consume Fox News programs (e.g., Gil de Zúñiga et al., 2012; Guess et al., 2021; Hmielowski et al., 2014; Iyengar & Hahn, 2009). On the contrary, outlets such as MSNBC and The *New York Times* were traditionally the Democrats' in-party source (Su et al., 2022) in that their stories "more closely matched the preferences of Democrats" (Iyengar & Hahn, 2009, p.24). Likewise, a bulk of studies has operationalized left-wing media utilization as how frequently people consume programs of MSNBC and so forth (e.g., Choi, 2022; Feldman et al., 2012; Hmielowski et al., 2022; Smith & Searles, 2014; Stroud, 2008).

Even though some prior research exhibited that the effects of partisan media consumption on public opinion might be limited (Guess et al., 2021), an overwhelming majority of studies in fact demonstrated that consuming partisan news can shape individuals' perceptions, attitudes, and behaviors (Levendusky, 2013), contributing to affective polarization and distrust in experts. Scholars have argued that since partisan media provide stories favoring a certain political side, it is hence highly possible that the given stories contain misleading information that benefit the aligned party, sow confusions, arouse hatred, or attack political opponents (Feldman et al., 2012; Bennett & Livingston, 2018; Hasell, 2021). As a result, audiences could become more likely to have affective repulsion toward their political counterparts and also become much more vulnerable to misinformation, disinformation, or false claims and statements featured in the partisan media they rely on (Kim & Kim, 2019; Weeks et al., 2021).

Unfortunately, many important health and environmental issues are politically fueled; hence, partisan media have inevitably influenced how these stories were told and how people subsequently perceive these issues (Chinn et al., 2020). For instance, one of the long-standing environmental issues, global warming, has become alarmingly politicized by the U.S. partisan media over the past decades (Chinn et al., 2020). Similarly, political polarization potentially driven by partisan media use also appeared amid the COVID-19 pandemic (e.g., Hart et al., 2020). Specifically, right-wing media oftentimes downplay the severity of the virus, referring to the COVID-19 as a hoax or a fraud (e.g., Halon, 2020). A poll before the 2020 U.S. Presidential Election precisely illustrated that nearly half of the U.S. voters hold the belief that the pandemic was "somewhat or mostly under control already" (Borah et al., 2022a, p. 5). Meanwhile, a panoply of research has also lent credence to a positive tie between conservative media use and misperceptions regarding public health crises such as the COVID-19 pandemic (Borah et al., 2022; Motta et al., 2020; Romer & Jamieson, 2020). On the contrary, liberal media were more likely to highlight the precautionary guidelines issued by health and governmental institutions and place more emphasis on the threats of the virus (Green et al., 2020).

Such a media divide is evidently reflected in public perceptions about the COVID-19. In terms of conservative media, for instance, Jamieson and Albarracine (2020) provided empirical evidence that COVID-19-related depictions and portrayals in conservative media outlets contained a variety of unfounded statements and unverified claims. Motta et al. (2020) revealed that people who frequently consume right-leaning media content were more likely to have conspiracy thinking and misperceptions about the COVID-19. Chung and Jones-Jang (2022) reported that utilizing Trump briefing and conservative outlets could reduce people's perceived severity of the pandemic, and thus decrease their willingness to abide by the recommended preventive measures amid the pandemic. When it comes to the role of liberal media use in influencing misperceptions, although the extant literature contains some mixed findings, most of them have suggested similarly positive effects (Garrett et al., 2016; Hmielowski et al., 2020; Weeks et al., 2021). The reasons are quite straightforward. As stated earlier, partisan media are committed to propagating ideas that are consistent with their political leanings and attack their political opponents (Garrett et al.,

2016); therefore, "facts oftentimes give way to predisposed ideologies and political interests" (Su et al., 2022, p. 3). To put it differently, partisan media's creating the "self-protective enclave of consistent messages" (p. 612) could effectively lead to the formation and crystallization of misperceptions among their viewers (Levendusky, 2013). Furthermore, the one-sided information typically contains more heuristic cues that help viewers to make sense of the reality hastily, also, these one-sided messages are oftentimes more "digestible" (p. 612) than those that entail multiple sources and mixed arguments (Levendusky, 2013) because the former could ease viewers' cognitive stresses, resulting in hasty formation of biased perceptions (Su et al., 2022).

2.1.3 Political Ideology

The influence of partisan media consumption on misperceptions does not occur equally among all individuals, instead, people's political ideology could serve as a factor upon which the effect is contingent. In other words, although it is widely confirmed that partisan media could facilitate the formation of misperceptions, the strength of such effect can still vary across people with different political ideologies (Amodio et al., 2007; Borah et al., 2023a; Federico & Goren, 2009). Therefore, I explore the moderating effect of my respondents' political ideology on the main association between partisan media consumption and the extent of their misperceptions regarding the COVID-19 pandemic.

Erikson and Tedin (2003) defined ideology as a "set of beliefs about the proper order of society and how it can be achieved" (p. 64). Denzau and North (1994) indicated that "ideologies are the shared framework of mental models that groups of individuals possess that provide both an interpretation of the environment and a prescription as to how that environment should be structured" (p. 24). When it comes to the impact of ideology, Jost and associates (2009) suggested that ideologies "crystallize and communicate the widely (but not unanimously) shared beliefs, opinions, and values of an identifiable group, class, constituency, or society" (p. 309). Moreover, ideologies can also depict the reality through making assertions or assumptions about human nature, historical events, present realities, and future possibilities," (p. 309) as well as "to envision the world as it should be, specifying acceptable means of attaining social, economic, and political ideals" (Jost et al., 2009, p. 309) Communication studies literature operationalize individuals' political ideology, in the U.S. context, as the extent to which they lean toward the liberal ideology or the conservative ideology according to their self-descriptions (Borah, 2022). A panoply of studies demonstrated that media effects could differ significantly across people at different positions in the ideological spectrum, and one's specific political ideology can even render the once significant media effect no longer competent in predicting psychological or behavioral responses (Borah et al., 2023a).

The theory of motivated reasoning describes exactly how individuals' political ideology could affect their perceptions (Bolsen et al., 2014; Leeper & Slothuus, 2014). Taber and Lodge (2006) indicated two primary motivations in information processing and perception forming, namely, directional goal and accuracy goal. In a nutshell, individuals seek information most likely congruent with their pre-existing views and beliefs while dismissing those at odds, and they regard these contents as accurate and credible (Druckman et al., 2013; Kunda, 1990; Lodge & Taber, 2005; Taber & Lodge, 2006). Strickland and associates (2011) aptly highlighted that citizens that are interested in politics and politically knowledgeable are oftentimes motivated to defend their pre-existing beliefs upon exposure to discrepant information. Such motivated reasoning process could further affect the ways in which individuals perceived public issues, policies, or specific social figures (Chaiken et al., 1996; Kunda, 1990; Strickland et al., 2011). Hence, politically motivated reasoning is extremely potent in driving misperceptions in that people with a strong partisan or ideological bias are not prone to be socially corrected even when they are exposed to corrective information or in a heterogeneous discussion network, rather, they would be more likely to defend the information congruent with their beliefs while attacking or intentionally circumventing those at odds.

In addition to the direct effect of political ideology, a plethora of studies has also lent sufficient credence to the moderating role of political ideology in shaping individuals' information processing, which in turn affects perception forming. For instance, Federico and Goren (2009) illustrated that ideology could be an "epistemic motivation" (p. 267) assisting individuals to situate themselves in the ideological spectrum, which in turn affects the ways in which they perceive the reality. This finding in fact resonates the assumption of motivated reasoning, suggesting how political ideology could indeed influence information processing and reality construction. Furthermore, Amodio and associates (2007) found that individuals self-identified as ideologically conservative were more persistent in their own judgements, while on the contrary, their liberal counterpart were more open to new experiences and exhibited greater tolerance to sophisticated information and situations. Likewise, Borah and colleagues (2023a) found significant moderating effects of political ideology. Specifically, they revealed that liberals with a greater level of media literacy for media content reported a lower level of COVID-19 misperceptions, however, this effect did not occur among conservatives. Similarly, Borah's (2022) survey study also showed that, against the research backdrop of the COVID-19 pandemic, the U.S. citizenships' political ideology significantly moderated the relationships between COVID-19 misperceptions and individuals' need for cognition, media locus of control, and misinformation efficacy.

I argue that exploring the role of American people's political ideology is particularly valuable because of the politicization of the pandemic (Green et al., 2020). The pandemic has already witnessed deep ideological divisions and profound affective polarization among the U.S. citizens (Druckman et al., 2021; Flores et al., 2022; Geiger et al., 2021). The Democrats and Republicans had deep discord and conflict on a series of the virus-related issues such as the very source of the virus, the effectiveness of the CDC recommended preventive measures, and even the authenticity of the virus (Jungkunz, 2021).

Meanwhile, the pandemic has also provided opportunities for the public to unleash, with the technological empowerment of social media, their hatred and disappointments toward the society, the government, the media, the elites, and so forth. This has led to the rampant circulation of misinformation, the proliferation of conspiracy theories, the deepening of xenophobia, and the erosion of the public trust in scientists. Regrettably, these are malign factors that intensify the structural conundrum of the post-truth era and undermine a healthy democratic society. Specific instances in this regard are extremely abundant. For example, Green et al. (2020) reported that liberals highlighted the specific threats that the pandemic poses to people's heath, whereas conservatives appeared to place more emphasis on political opponents and economy. A great deal of evidence also demonstrates that in the U.S., Republicans tend to perceive that the pandemic is not as severe, such that they themselves are not willing to engage in protective measurements, while Democrats relied more on experts' sources and had a much greater risk perception (Allcott et al., 2020; Gadarian et al., 2021; Green et al., 2020). Moreover, the then-president Donald Trump has been called "the largest driver of the infodemic" (Stolberg & Wieland, 2020) due to he constant promotion of misinformation and conspiracy theories (Carey et al., 2022). Hatch (2020) argued that Trump's communications through mass media and social media platforms have contributed to the polarization of the country. More worryingly, plenty of studies have shown that those who relied heavily on Trump for COVID-19 information exhibited greater misperceptions (e.g., Druckman et al., 2021; Borah et al., 2023a; Mitchell et al., 2021). Building upon these studies, it is safe to say that the political ideology of U.S. citizens could affect their misperceptions with respect to the pandemic.

2.1.4 Need for Cognition

In addition to individuals' political ideology, I take a step further to investigate whether need for cognition (NFC) could be another condition upon which the effects of partisan media use on misperceptions regarding the COVID-19 pandemic is contingent. NFC is "a stable personality trait that describes individuals' tendency to engage in and enjoy effortful cognitive activity" (Lins de Holanda Coelho et al., 2020, p. 1870). In communication research, NFC usually represents the extent to which people prefer actively, consciously, effortfully, and logically processing information that they are exposed to (Austin et al., 2016). According to Cacioppo and Petty (1982), NFC is statistical rather than biological, and NFC-oriented people are prone to engage in critical thinking. On the contrary, non-NFC-oriented individuals usually rely on the heuristic processing approach to make sense of the information they are exposed to (Austin et al., 2016; Su et al., 2021). However, this heuristic processing approach requires less cognitive efforts. For the most part, NFC is seen as tightly related to media literacy (Cacioppo & Petty, 1982; Epstein et al., 1996; Huber et al., 2022; Koc & Barut, 2016; Su et al., 2021; Xiao et al., 2021b).

A high-level NFC could prevent individuals from falling for misinformation and going astray. Extant literature has rendered rich evidence to bolster the negative impact of NFC on people's misperceptions. In their experimental study, Leding and Antonio (2019) showed that individuals who had a high score on NFC were "less susceptible" to misinformation (p. 409). Su et al. (2021) showed that NFC was negatively associated with COVID-19 misperceptions. Likewise, Borah's (2022) survey research demonstrated that individuals who scored higher on NFC exhibited lower COVID-19 misperceptions. Xiao and associates (2021b) found that NFC was a positive predictor of individuals' critical consuming literacy, which in turn tied negatively to misperceptions regarding HPV vaccines.

Additionally, NFC also has the potential to function as a moderator in various contexts. Vafeiadis and Xiao (2021) performed an experiment investigating the interplay of consumer involvement, NFC, and emotional reactions when participants are exposed to social media fake news. Their study revealed that people who scored higher on NFC perceived the rebuttal message more favorably and exhibited positive attitudes when it responded to the rumors. Tsfati and Cappella (2005) found that NFC moderated the association between news exposure and media skepticism. That is, among those with higher NFC, the once significant tie between news exposure and media skepticism disappeared. In researching on misperceptions, the moderating role of NFC is also found. Su et al. (2021) suggested that among Chinese people, NFC moderated the indirect association between international social media use and conspiracy theory endorsement of COVID-19 through media skepticism. In other words, among those with a higher level of NFC, the indirect effect became more negative. In this case, NFC buffered the role of social media use in shaping conspiracy beliefs, lending credence to its relationship with critical consuming media literacy (Xiao et al., 2021b). Following the reviewed literature, I posit that NFC could moderate the association between partisan media use and COVID-19 misperceptions. In other words, I postulate that among those who favor critical, logical, and statistical processing of information, the effect of partisan media use on misperceptions is expected to be reduced.

2.1.5 Trust in Scientists

As mentioned earlier, motivated reasoning functions conditionally instead of pervasively, in addition to individuals' political ideology and need for cognition, I also examine whether their trust in scientists would moderate the effect of partisan media use on misperceptions. Trust and faith can mitigate "ideologically driven endorsement of misinformation" (Miller et al., 2016, p. 827). Studies have shown that trust can moderate the effects of communication on perceptions, beliefs, attitudes, and behaviors (Ardèvol-Abreu et al., 2018; Miller et al., 2016). This vein of research is diversified in terms of study context. Prior studies have investigated the role of trust in political institutions, media organization, information sources, and media ownerships (Williams, 2012).

For instance, defined as "a summary judgment that the system is responsive and will do what is right even in the absence of constant scrutiny" (Miller & Listhaug, 1990, p. 358), trust in political systems can buttress the functioning of democracy and moderate the role of media use in shaping civic engagement and political participation (Su & Xiao, 2022). This is because if "individuals in the system are not sufficiently oriented toward one another" (McLaren, 2012, p. 165), political systems are likely to fail. When it comes to the trust in media, scholars found that it can function as a motivational characteristic of media viewers, directing them to allocate more cognitive resources to those they trust while circumventing those they distrust.

People's expectations of social trust are stemmed from "commonly shared values" (Ardèvol-Abreu et al., 2018, p. 614), either in the form of "deep values" or more secular principles such as "professional standards and codes of behavior" (Fukuyama, 1995, p. 26). A certain extent of trust is deemed imperative in not only building a cohesive society but also in facilitating healthy interpersonal interactions and discussions (Eisenstadt et al., 1984; Tsfati & Cappella, 2003). According to Goodwin and Jasper (2006), bonds of trust among "members of a social movement" could help constitute collective identity (p. 617). This argument should also apply to trust in scientists and experts amid the COVID-19 pandemic. Against the backdrop that the pandemic has deeply intensified the affective polarization among the U.S. citizens, trust in scientists could help constitute a shared identity among some individuals, which in turn creates mutual encouragement to follow scientific discourse among them. In the current post-truth era, the credibility and persuasiveness of expert discourse has been severely challenged. Not only do individuals have enough information sources to choose freely, but they can even be provided with a pseudo-environment constructed by algorithm, which satisfies most of their information needs. In this case, expert discourses have encountered huge obstacles in forming direct and powerful dissemination effects, after all, the very purpose of dissemination is audiences' acceptance. Professionals and pundits are still at the end of their tether in the face of their declining credibility, hence, a factor that varies the effects is the extent to which people trust in scientists.

In this section, I include trust in scientists as another moderator, examining whether the extent to which individuals' trust in scientists could vary the effects of partisan media use on COVID-19 misperceptions. Despite exposure to partisan media such as Fox News and MSNBC, people's high level of trust in scientists may hinder the independent variable (i.e., consuming partisan media) from eroding their faith system or prevent them from falling for misinformation.

2.1.6 Message Derogation

The effect of partisan media use on misperceptions might exert indirectly, in other words, exposure to partisan media may not necessarily lead to misperceptions immediately, instead, it may function through initially shaping some specific attitudes that further catalyse the crystallization of false beliefs, constituting a mediating mechanism. One such mediating factor pertains to individuals' derogatory attitudes toward COVID-19 related news and information on mass media. The concept of message derogation stems from the Extended Parallel Process Model (EPPM). According to the EPPM (Witte, 1992), individuals tend to reduce fear when perceived threat is high and perceived efficacy is low. Two commonly studied approaches of fear control are defensive avoidance and news derogation (Roberto et al., 2021; Stephenson & Witte, 1998).

Defensive avoidance involves conscious efforts in avoiding specific messages or scenarios, such as leaving a specific webpage, ignoring a conversation, or changing the channel to prevent exposure to some specific information (McMahan et al., 1998). News derogation refers to the derogatory attitudes toward or reactions to disgust about the news on media, which is oftentimes manifested by behaviors such as criticizing the specific message or the source of the message (Hong, 2011). In the context of the COVID-19, for instance, news derogation is reflected in the belief that the relevant news exaggerates the threat of the pandemic (Popova, 2012; Witte, 1994, 1998a). In terms of its operationalization, news derogation has been measured by the extent to which individuals perceive the news information or messages they are exposed to as exaggerated, distorted, overstated, exploitative, misleading, or manipulative (e.g., Su et al., 2022; Thompson et al., 2011). In this section, I include derogation of COVID-19 related messages on mass media as a mediator between partisan media use and COVID-19 misperception. Specifically, I posit that using partisan media would first result in either an increase or a decrease in derogatory attitudes toward COVID-19 related news on non-partisan mass media, which in turn influences the formation of misperceptions.

In terms of using partisan media during the COVID-19 pandemic, scholars argued that using conservative media triggers rejection and demeaning of the news media (e.g., Conway III et al., 2021). This is because conservative media viewers are oftentimes hostile to the pandemic, "have greater perceived pressure for change" (Su et al., 2022, p. 5), and believe those objectively depicted stories threaten their agency and freedoms (Thrasher et al., 2016). When it comes to liberal media use, the effect might be the opposite, as liberal media such as MSNBC were prone to convey plenty of scientific sources such as medical experts and scientists, hence, liberal media viewers would have a greater perceived susceptibility and severity, engaging more actively in scientists-recommended preventive measures (Chung & Jones-Jang, 2022; Jamieson & Albarracine, 2020; Moon et al., 2022; Su et al., 2022).

2.1.7 Moderated Mediation Models

To sum up, this chapter entails the following examinations. First, I explore the main relationships between Fox News and MSNBC use and COVID-19 misperceptions. In addition to the main associations between partisan media use and misperceptions regarding COVID-19, I investigate three moderation effects, namely, whether individuals' political ideology, need for cognition, and trust in scientists could moderate the main relationships. I posit that the influence of partisan media use would not exert equally among people, instead, it would function conditionally according to the three moderating factors.

Next, I include message derogation as a mediator, the purpose is to probe whether exposing to Fox News and MSNBC would influence people's derogatory attitude toward COVID-19 prior to leading to the formation of misperceptions. Lastly, I integrate the moderators and the mediator in the main effect, exploring three moderated mediation models. In all models, Fox News use and MSNBC use are the two independent variables, misperceptions regarding COVID-19 is the dependent variable, and message derogation is the mediator. The three models contain three moderators, which function at the path between partisan media use and message derogation.

2.2 Methodology

2.2.1 Data Collection

After approval of the IRB at the university in which the author was affiliated, this survey study was administered through a questionnaire on Qualtrics, and the fieldwork as conducted in October 2021. The author utilized the Amazon Mechanical Turk to recruit participants. Amazon MTurk has been extensively utilized for sampling, which is considered an ideal platform to collect more geographically diversified and politically representative data and to offer a credible source of respondents for studies that aim at examining cognitive processes of human beings instead of inferring general population estimates (Amazeen, 2020; Berinsky et al., 2012; Boas et al., 2020). That being said, it warrants noticing that MTurk might not always provide a substitute for population-based samples. Respondents were people that resided in the United States at the time the survey was conducted. Moreover, only those above the age of 18 were recruited. Each participant was compensated with 1.1 dollar. As a result, 1004 individuals took part in the survey. Upon collection of the initial data, the author removed incomplete sample, rendering 915 samples. These samples are the final valid samples sent for analysis.

2.2.2 Measurements

COVID-19 misperceptions. The measurement of the COVID-19 misperceptions consists of nine items. Each item was a piece of misinformation or conspiracy theory, and the respondents were asked to indicate the extent to which they agreed with each statement on a 5-point Likert scale (1 = strongly disagree, 5 = strongly agree). The statements include "COVID-19 death rates are inflated," "Wearing a mask does not protect you from COVID-19," "5G radiant is the real cause of COVID-19," "Bill Gates intends to implant microchips in people via COVID-19 vaccination," and so forth. It warrants noticing that misinformation and conspiracy theories do not necessarily mean that the message is fake, it highlights that the information per se lacks any scientific evidence and can facilitate the devastation of the "infodemic" (Himelboim et al., 2023). The measurement of this variable reached satisfactory internal reliability ($M = 3.47$, $SD = 1.09$, $\alpha = 0.95$).

Fox News use. Fox News use is measured by the frequencies with which the respondents consume news through the Fox News channel on a 5-point Likert scale (1 = never, 5 = always; $M = 3.57$, $SD = 1.22$).

MSNBC News use. MSNBC News use is assessed by the frequencies with which the participants consume news through MSNBC on a 5-point Likert scale (1 = never, 5 = always; $M = 3.61$, $SD = 1.12$).

Political ideology. Political ideology is measured through asking the respondent to answer the following question on a 5-point Likert scale (1 = very conservative, 5 = very liberal), "Which of the following best describes your political ideology?" ($M = 2.54$, $SD = 1.38$).

Trust in scientists. Trust in scientists is measured by asking the respondents to answer, on a 5-point Likert scale (1 = not at all, 5 = a great deal), the following question, "How much you trust scientists as a source of information about COVID-19?" ($M = 2.03$, $SD = 0.97$).

Need for cognition. Need for cognition is evaluated by asking the respondents to indicate the extent to which they agree with the following six statements, "I would prefer complex to simple problems," "I like to have the responsibility of handling a situation that requires a lot of thinking," "Thinking is not my idea of fun," "I would rather do something that requires little thought than something that is sure to challenge my thinking abilities," "I really enjoy a task that involves coming up with new solutions to problems," and "I would prefer a task that is intellectual, difficult, and important to one that is somewhat important but does not require much thought" via a 5-point Likert scale (1 = strongly disagree, 5 = strongly agree) The third and fourth items were reverse coded to keep consistency ($M = 3.47$, $SD = 1.09$, $\alpha = 0.72$).

COVID-19 message derogation. Message derogation of COVID-19 is measured by comprising four items. The respondents were asked to indicate the extent to which they agree that the information about the COVID-19 provided by the mass media is "exaggerated," "manipulated," "distorted," and "overblown" via a 5-point Likert scale (1 = strongly disagree, 5 = strongly agree; $M = 3.63$, $SD = 1.08$, $\alpha = 0.91$).

Control variables. In addition to the endogenous variables, I also added control variables into the models to remove the concern of spurious effects. The respondents were first asked to report their age in numeric form ($M = 37.47$, $SD = 11.07$). The respondents' gender was also measured through a dummy variable (44% female, 56% male). The respondent' race was also surveyed (79.5% White, 20.5% non-whites). The respondents' education level was administered by their self-reported educational degrees (*Median* = 5 [Bachelor's degree], $SD = 0.83$), monthly income (*Median* = 4 [$8000-$10,000], $SD = 1.61$). Given the fact that the pandemic has been significantly politicized in United States, the respondents' Party ID was controlled. Party ID was measured on a 5-point Likert scale (1 = strong Republican, 5 = strong Democrat; M = 3.29, SD = 1.53). Additionally, the respondents' interests in news and politics were also added as control variables. News interest and political interest were measured by asking the respondents to rate their interests in news and politics in a 5-point Likert scale, respectively (1 = not at all interested, 5 = extremely interested; M_{news} = 3.90, SD_{news} = 1.06; $M_{politics}$ = 3.71, $SD_{politics}$ = 1.07).

2.2.3 Analytical Strategy

To examine the direct effects of partisan media use on COVID-19 misperceptions, I use hierarchical regression. In terms of the moderation effects of political ideology, NFC, and trust in scientists, Hayes' (2018) PROCESS macro model 1 was applied. To investigate the mediating role of COVID-19 message derogation, I applied Hayes' (2018) PROCESS macro model 4. When it comes to the moderated mediation effects, PROCESS macro model 7 was performed.

2.3 Results

First, as can be seen in Table 2.1, it is found that beyond all controls, the use of Fox News is positively associated with misperceptions of COVID-19 (b = 0.519, SE = 0.022, p < .001), implying that the more people consume news from the Fox News, the more likely they fall for the misinformation regarding the COVID-19 pandemic and have greater misperceptions. Similarly, as Table 2.2 shows, there is also a significant positive association between MSNBC news use and COVID-19 related misperceptions (b = 0.364, SE = 0.026, p < .001), implying that consuming news through MSNBC channel can also facilitate beliefs in COVID-19 misperceptions.

In addition to the main associations, I also analysed the moderation effects using PROCESS macro model 1, aiming to understand whether political ideology, NFC, and trust in scientists can moderate the main relationships between Fox News use, MSNBC use, and COVID-19 misperceptions. First and foremost, controlling for all covariates, the result of the 95% bias-corrected confidence intervals from 5,000 bootstrapped samples demonstrated that the main association between Fox News use and COVID-19 misperceptions was significantly moderated by the respondents' political ideology (b = 0.1263, *Boot SE* = 0.141, t = 8.9492, p < .001, 95% CI = [0.0986, 0.1540]). Figure 2.1 visualizes the interaction effect. As can be seen in Figure 2.1, among those leaning liberal, the effect of Fox News use on COVID-19 misperceptions became stronger (*Effect* = 0.5796, SE = 0.0240, t = 24.1173, p < .001, 95% CI = [0.5324, 0.6267]), compared to those neutral (*Effect* = 0.3270, SE = 0.0275, t = 11.8837, p < .001, 95% CI = [0.2730, 0.3811]) and those leaning conservative (*Effect* = 0.2008, SE = 0.380, t = 5.2826, p < .001, 95% CI = [0.1262, 0.2754]). When it comes to the moderating role of political ideology in shaping the associations between

Table 2.1 Main direct effects of Fox New use on COVID-19 misperceptions

	COVID-19 Misperceptions		
Step 1	*b*	*SE*	*t*
Constant	4.844***	0.256	18.902
Age	−0.008**	0.003	0.290
Gender	−0.421***	−0.192	−6.823
Race	−0.250***	0.023	−10.744
Education	−0.230***	0.044	−5.250
Monthly income	0.273***	0.021	13.038
Party ID	−0.109***	0.021	−5.128
News interest	0.111**	0.041	2.702
Political interest	0.025	0.040	0.606
R^2	0.303***		
Step 2			
Constant	2.462***	0.227	10.850
Age	−0.001	0.002	−0.583
Gender	−0.172**	0.050	−3.446
Race	−0.136***	0.019	−7.131
Education	−0.129***	0.035	−3.696
Income	0.182***	0.017	10.680
Party ID	−0.044*	0.017	−2.557
News interest	−0.005	0.033	00.142
Political interest	−0.040	0.032	−1.238
Fox News Use	0.519***	0.022	23.265
R^2	0.566***		

Notes: Cell entries (b) are unstandardized betas. SE: Standard error. *$p < .05$, **$p < .01$, ***$p < .001$.

Table 2.2 Main direct effects of MSNBC use on COVID-19 misperceptions

	COVID-19 Misperceptions		
Step 1	*b*	*SE*	*t*
Constant	3.560***	0.265	13.423
Age	−0.009**	0.003	−3.330
Gender	−0.227***	0.060	−3.757
Race	−0.171***	0.023	−7.453
Education	−0.060	0.044	−1.361
Monthly income	0.245***	0.020	12.295
Party ID	−0.094***	0.020	−4.694
News interest	0.116**	0.039	2.976
Political interest	0.058	0.039	1.524
R^2	0.262		
Step 2			
Constant	2.869***	0.245	11.690
Age	−0.005	0.002	−1.857
Gender	−0.219***	0.055	−4.000
Race	−0.143	0.021	−6.852
Education	−0.107**	0.040	−2.699

(*Continued*)

Table 2.2 (Continued)

	COVID-19 Misperceptions		
Step 1	*b*	*SE*	*t*
Income	0.188***	0.019	10.177
Party ID	−0.105***	0.018	−5.777
News interest	0.054	0.035	1.535
Political interest	0.025	0.035	0.708
MSNBC News Use	0.364***	0.026	13.784
R^2	0.395		

Notes: Cell entries (b) are unstandardized betas. SE: Standard error. *$p < .05$, **$p < .01$, ***$p < .001$.

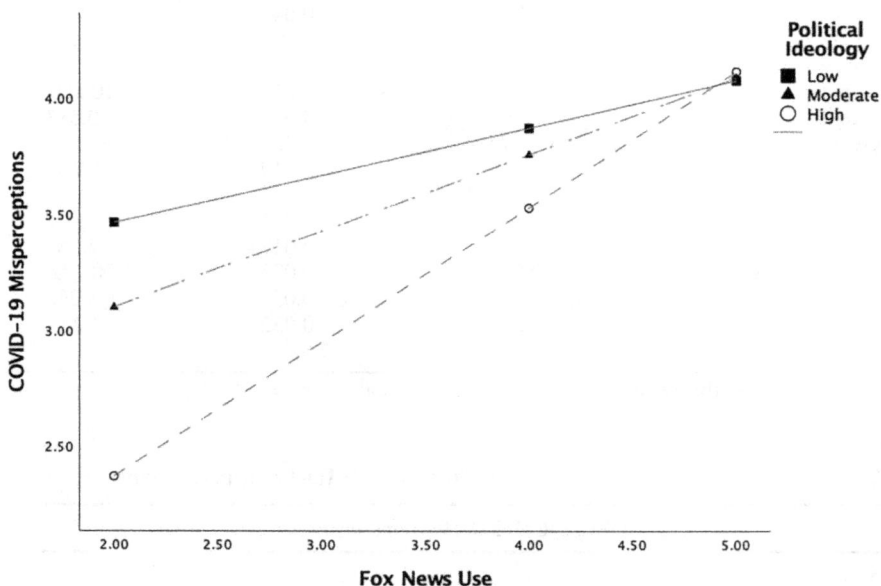

Figure 2.1 Two-way interaction between Fox News use and political ideology on COVID-19 misperceptions.

MSNBC use and COVID-19 misperceptions, controlling for all covariates, the result of the 95% bias-corrected confidence intervals from 5,000 bootstrapped samples demonstrated that the main association between MSNBC News use and COVID-19 misperceptions was significantly moderated by individuals' political ideology ($b = 0.110$, *Boot SE* = 0.016, $t = 6.736$, $p < .001$, 95% CI = [0.0778, 0.1417]). Figure 2.2 visualizes the interaction effect. Specifically, among those reported leaning liberal, the effect of MSNBC news use on COVID-19 misperceptions became stronger (*Effect* = 0.5014, *SE* = 0.0340, $t = 14.7300$, $p < .001$, 95% CI = [0.4346, 0.5682]), compared to those neutral (*Effect* = 0.2819, *SE* = 0.0267, $t = 10.5444$, $p < .001$, 95% CI = [0.2294, 0.3344])

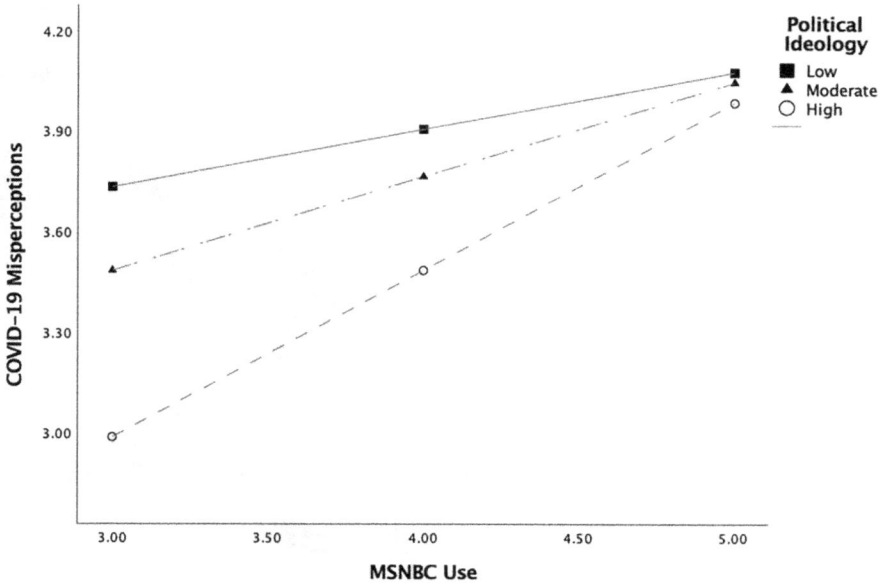

Figure 2.2 Two-way interaction between MSNBC news use and political ideology on COVID-19 misperceptions.

and those leaning conservative (*Effect* = 0.1722, *SE* = 0.359, *t* = 4.7954, *p* < .001, 95% CI = [0.1017, 0.2427]).

I also applied the same analysis to examine whether NFC can moderate the main effects of Fox News use and MSNBC use on COVID-19 misperceptions. First, controlling for all covariates, the result of the 95% bias-corrected confidence intervals from 5,000 bootstrapped samples demonstrated that the main association between Fox News use and COVID-19 misperceptions was not moderated by individuals' NFC (*b* = 0.0099, *Boot SE* = 0.319, *t* = 0.3085, *p* = 0.7577, 95% CI = [−0.0528, 0.0725]). However, when it comes to the moderating role of NFC in shaping the associations between MSNBC news use and COVID-19 misperceptions, controlling for all covariates, the result of the 95% bias-corrected confidence intervals from 5,000 bootstrapped samples demonstrated that the main association between MSNBC News use and COVID-19 misperceptions was significantly moderated by individuals' degrees of NFC (*b* = −0.1925, *Boot SE* = 0.0388, *t* = −4.9659, *p* < .001, 95% CI = [−0.2686, −0.1164]). Figure 2.3 visualizes the interaction effect. Specifically, among those reported higher NFC, the effect of MSNBC news use on COVID-19 misperceptions became weaker (*Effect* = 0.2760, *SE* = 0.0314, *t* = 8.7894, *p* < .001, 95% CI = [0.2143, 0.3376]), compared to those with a moderate level of NFC (*Effect* = 0.3722, *SE* = 0.0255, *t* = 14.6109, *p* < .001, 95% CI = [0.3222, 0.4222]) and those with lower level of NFC (*Effect* = 0.4364, *SE* = 0.0290, *t* = 15.0400, *p* < .001, 95% CI = [0.3794, 0.4933]).

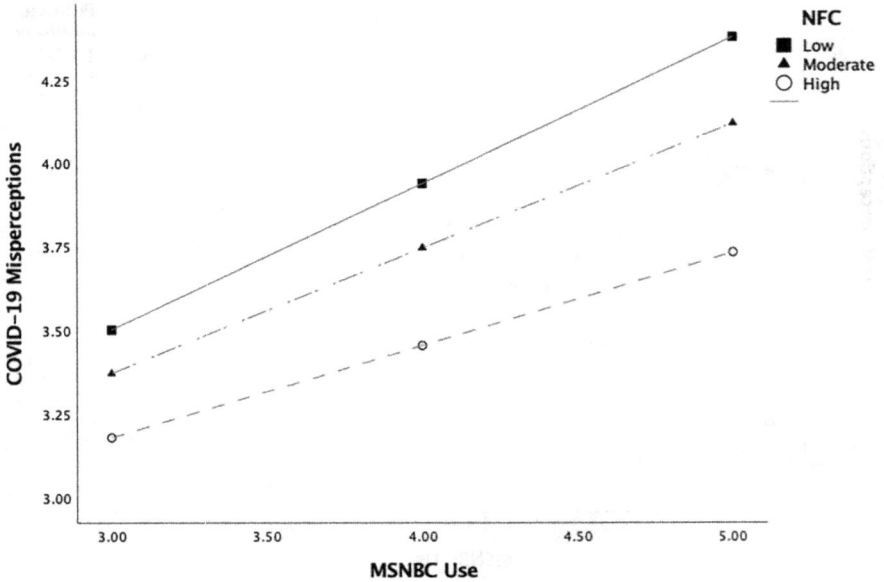

Figure 2.3 Two-way interaction between MSNBC use and NFC on COVID-19 misperceptions.

Same moderation analysis was performed to investigate the role of trust in scientists in moderating the main direct effects of Fox News use and MSNBC news use on COVID-19 misperceptions. First, controlling for all covariates, the result of the 95% bias-corrected confidence intervals from 5,000 bootstrapped samples demonstrated that the main association between Fox News use and COVID-19 misperceptions was significantly moderated by individuals' trust in scientists ($b = -0.1541$, *Boot SE* $= 0.0193$, $t = -7.9961$, $p < .001$, 95% CI $= [0.1920, 0.1163]$). Figure 2.4 visualizes the interaction effect. Specifically, among those reported greater trust in scientists, the effect of Fox News use on COVID-19 misperceptions became weaker (*Effect* $= 0.3534$, *SE* $= 0.0300$, $t = 11/7778$, $p < .001$, 95% CI $= [0.2945, 0.4123]$), compared to those with moderate level of trust (*Effect* $= 0.5076$, *SE* $= 0.0215$, $t = 23.5751$, $p < .001$, 95% CI $= [0.4653, 0.5498]$) and those with lower level of trust in scientists (*Effect* $= 0.6617$, *SE* $= 0.0277$, $t = 23.8520$, $p < .001$, 95% CI $= [0.6073, 0.7162]$).

When it comes to the moderating role of trust in scientists in affecting the association between MSNBC use and COVID-19 misperceptions, controlling for all covariates, the result of the 95% bias-corrected confidence intervals from 5,000 bootstrapped samples demonstrated that the main association between MSNBC use and COVID-19 misperceptions was significantly moderated by individuals' trust in scientists ($b = -0.0943$, *Boot SE* $= 0.0214$, $t =$

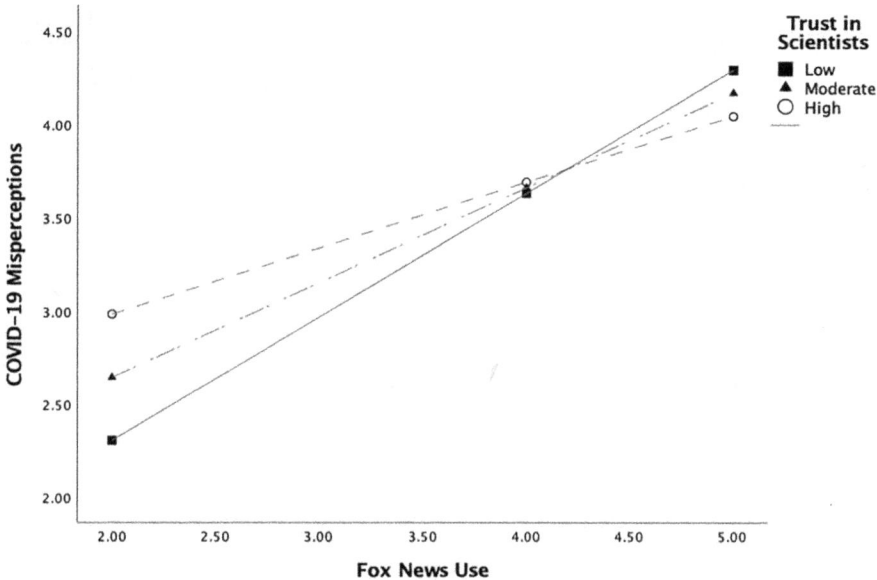

Figure 2.4 Two-way interaction between Fox News use and trust in scientists on COVID-19 misperceptions.

−4.4032, $p < .001$, 95% CI = [−0.1363, −0.0523]). Figure 2.5 visualizes the interaction effect. Specifically, among those reported higher level of trust in scientists, the effect of MSNBC news use on COVID-19 misperceptions became weaker (*Effect* = 0.3131, *SE* = 0.0306, $t = 10.2307$, $p < .001$, 95% CI = [0.2530, 0.3731]), compared to those with a moderate level of trust (*Effect* = 0.4073, *SE* = 0.0270, $t = 15.0898$, $p < .001$, 95% CI = [0.3544, 0.4603]) and those with a lower level of trust in scientists (*Effect* = 0.5016, *SE* = 0.379, $t = 13.2274$, $p < .001$, 95% CI = [0.4272, 0.5761]).

Next, I analyzed the mediating role of message derogation. First, in terms of the indirect effect of Fox News use on COVID-19 misperceptions, the result of the Hayes' (2018) PROCESS macro model 4 showed that the mediation model is significant (*Effect* = 0.2940, *Boot SE* = 0.0230, 95% CI = [0.2504, 0.3404]). Specifically, using Fox News is positively associated with message derogation of COVID-19 ($b = 0.4504$, *SE* = 0.2460, $t = 18.3434$, $p < .001$, 95% CI = [0.4022, 0.4986]), which in turn led to greater COVID-19 misperceptions ($b = 0.6528$, *SE* = 0.0211, $t = 30.9373$, $p < .001$, 95% CI = [0.6114, 0.6942]). Next, when it comes to the indirect effect of MSNBC news use on COVID-19 misperceptions, the result of the Hayes' (2018) PROCESS macro model 4 also demonstrated that the mediation model is significant (*Effect* = 0.1715, *Boot SE* = 0.0258, 95% CI = [0.1214, 0.2233]). Specifically, using MSNBC is positively associated with message derogation of COVID-19 ($b = 0.2449$, *SE* = 0.0282,

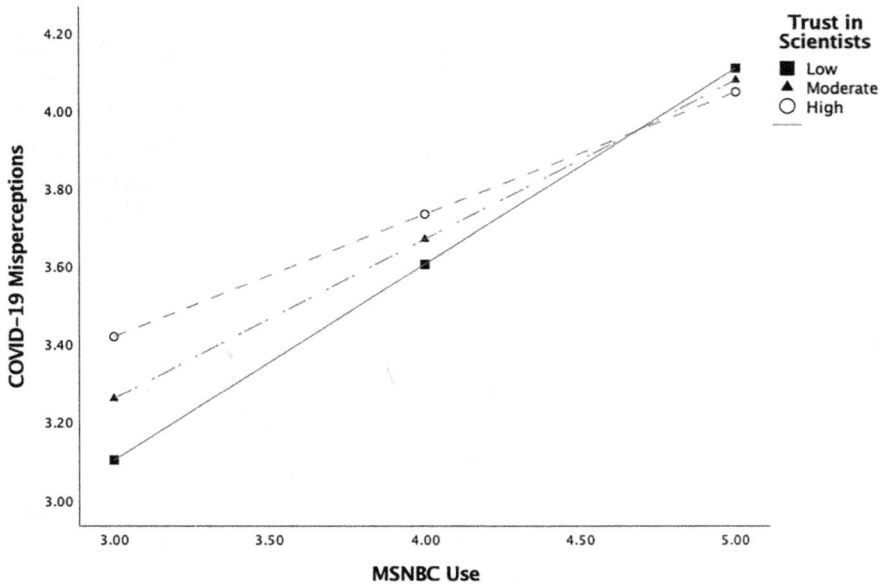

Figure 2.5 Two-way interaction between MSNBC news use and trust in scientists on COVID-19 misperceptions.

$t = 8.6691$, $p < .001$, 95% CI = [0.1894, 0.3003]), which in turn led to greater COVID-19 misperceptions ($b = 0.7004$, $SE = 0.0211$, $t = 33.2620$, $p < .001$, 95% CI = [0.6590, 0.7417]).

As I have stated earlier, another goal of this section is to unpack conditional indirect effects of partisan media use on COVID-19 misperceptions, hence, I ran six moderated mediation models. The moderated mediation models were analyzed by Hayes' (2018) PROCESS macro model 7, which further demonstrated how political ideology, NFC, and trust in scientists vary the indirect effects. First, the model exhibited that political ideology significantly moderated the association between Fox News use and COVID-19 misperceptions that is mediated through message derogation (*Moderated mediation index* = 0.0661, *Boot SE* = 0.0123, 95% CI = [0.0423, 0.0908]). Specifically, the bootstrapped 95% bias-corrected confidence intervals suggest that the positive effect of Fox News use on COVID-19 misperceptions mediated through message derogation became stronger among those with greater liberal ideology ($b = 0.3296$, *Boot SE* = .0.0259, 95% CI = [0.2796, 0.3818]) compared to those with neutral ($b = 0.1975$, *Boot SE* = .0.0246, 95% CI = [0.1484, 0.2464]) and greater conservative ideology ($b = 0.1314$, *Boot SE* = .0.0321, 95% CI = [0.0670, 0.1938]).

Moreover, the model illustrated that political ideology also significantly moderated the association between MSNBC news use and COVID-19 misperception that is mediated through message derogation (*Moderated mediation index* = 0.0629, *Boot SE* = 0.0150, 95% CI = [0.0339, 0.0922]). Specifically, the bootstrapped 95% bias-corrected confidence intervals suggest that the positive effect of MSNBC news use on COVID-19 misperceptions mediated through message derogation became stronger among those with greater liberal ideology (*b* = 0.2540, *Boot SE* = .0.0344, 95% CI = [0.1889, 0.3229]) compared to those with neutral (*b* = 0.1282, *Boot SE* = .0.0263, 95% CI = [0.0773, 0.1816]) and greater conservative ideology (*b* = 0.0653, *Boot SE* = .0.0334, 95% CI = [0.0006, 0.1317]).

Next, the same analyses were applied to examine whether NFC can moderate the indirect effects. The model illustrated that the association between Fox News use and COVID-19 misperception that is mediated through message derogation was varied by NFC (*Moderated mediation index* = 0.0986, *Boot SE* = 0.0387, 95% CI = [0.0250, 0.1781]). Specifically, the bootstrapped 95% bias-corrected confidence intervals suggest that the positive effect of Fox news use on COVID-19 misperceptions mediated through message derogation became stronger among those with greater NFC (*b* = 0.2985, *Boot SE* = .0.0233, 95% CI = [0.2527, 0.3443]) compared to those with moderate (*b* = 0.2492, *Boot SE* = .0.0246, 95% CI = [0.2009, 0.2963]) and lower NFC (*b* = 0.2164, *Boot SE* = .0.0326, 95% CI = [0.1519, 0.2800]). However, when it comes to the indirect effect of MSNBC news use on COVID-19 misperceptions, NFC was not a significant moderate (*Moderated mediation index* = −0.0848, *Boot SE* = 0.0467, 95% CI = [−0.1754, 0.0076]).

Finally, I ran the model to investigate whether the extent of trust in scientists can also be a condition upon which the indirect effects of partisan media use on COVID-19 misperceptions are contingent. In terms of the Fox News use, the model suggested that the indirect effects of Fox News use on COVID-19 misperception mediated through message derogation was moderated by trust in scientists (*Moderated mediation index* = −0.1227, *Boot SE* = 0.0186, 95% CI = [0.1606, 0.0867]). Specifically, the bootstrapped 95% bias-corrected confidence intervals suggest that the positive effect of Fox News use on COVID-19 misperceptions mediated through message derogation became weaker among those with greater trust in scientists (*b* = 0.1624, *Boot SE* = .0.0304, 95% CI = [0.1012, 0.2201]) compared to those with moderate (*b* = 0.2851, *Boot SE* = .0.0222, 95% CI = [0.2426, 0.3285]) and lower degrees of trust (*b* = 0.4078, *Boot SE* = .0.0275, 95% CI = [0.3544, 0.4615]). When it comes to the indirect effect of MSNBC news use on COVID-19 misperceptions, I found that trust in scientists was also a significant moderator (*Moderated mediation index* = −0.1042, *Boot SE* = 0.0210, 95% CI = [−0.1456, −0.0634]). Specifically, the bootstrapped 95% bias-corrected confidence intervals illustrate that the positive effect of MSNBC news use on COVID-19 misperceptions mediated through message derogation became weaker among those with greater trust in scientists (*b* = 0.1088, *Boot SE* = .0.0311, 95% CI = [0.0478, 0.1686]) compared to those with moderate (*b* = 0.2130, *Boot SE* = .0.0242, 95% CI = [0.1661, 0.2615]) and lower degrees of trust (*b* = 0.3173, *Boot SE* = .0.0329, 95% CI = [0.2517, 0.3830]).

2.4 Conclusion and Discussion

Pundits have long lamented that vast misinformation and conspiracy theories would undermine the bedrock of a democratic society. The chaos caused by misinformation amid the COVID-19 pandemic is a vivid example of such argument. Miscellaneous sources of information have resulted in a loss of guidance, worthwhile for relying on among citizens; while the current high-choice information environment, individuals' gradually formed ambient awareness, and their passive news consumptive strategy have also significantly empowered algorithmic mechanism to construct realities and further power-fully shape people's perceptions and attitudes. Various societal issues, including the decline in the credibility of government agencies and expert groups, have made people no longer trust the discourses of authorities and scientific communities, and become more susceptible to conspiracy theories that either fit their own pre-existing ideology or are charged with storytelling narratives and characteristics that enhances its appeal and persuasiveness. As far as the communication research is concerned, a great deal of research has been de-voted to examining what kind of sources lead to the proliferation of misinfor-mation and the crystallization of misperceptions. Although the COVID-19 pandemic is still a rather novel research topic, the evidence in this regard seems to be quite detailed, comprehensive, and solid. Of course, the unique phenomenon of "infodemic" was formed in this social media era. Therefore, the dissemination characteristics of social media information are the main driving force, and abundant research results have consistently confirmed this point.

That being said, traditional mass media still cannot stay aloof. Indeed, par-tisan media outlets have facilitated the spread of misinformation and conspir-acy theories, even playing the role of the culprit (Xiao et al., 2021). Major partisan media outlets not only straightforwardly influence their audiences through their strong agenda-setting influence but also provide a large number of initial sources for accounts on social media platforms, giving rise to various alternative spaces for the dissemination of misinformation and disinformation. Partisan media are committed to facilitating certain agendas and systemati-cally triggering misperceptions consistent with the interest of their affiliated party or even politicians. For instance, Fox News not only "constituted an echo chamber that promoted and defended conservativism" (Su et al., 2022, p. 3) but also, during the COVID-19 pandemic, became a vocal supporter of the Donald Trump, advancing his discourses that the pandemic is a hoax while urging the opposite of his medical experts who had been pleading caution.

Against this backdrop, this section examines and discusses the conditional indirect effects of using two partisan media, Fox News and MSNBC, on COVID-19 misperceptions. The results showed that using both Fox News and MSNBC tied to increased misperceptions about COVID-19. As for the posi-tive effect of Fox News use on misperceptions, it comes as no surprise, while what is a bit unexpected was the similarly positive effect of MSNBC on misperceptions. In fact, as I have stated in the above literature review section, the extent to which liberal media use could affect misperceptions is often case-sensitive, which explains why plenty of prior empirical studies have drawn mixed, and even conflicting conclusions. As far as the COVID-19 pandemic is concerned, liberal media did tend to include more scientists' claims in their news coverage than their conservative counterpart. However, when we consider the international nature of the pandemic per se, it is safe to say that the liberal and conservative media in the United States have unanimously held an anti-China stance (Galston, 2021). More specifically, the issue of the origin of the virus had been used as an ideal excuse to divert the U.S. domestic conflicts amid its 2016 election. Trump and his conservative media allies had always been committed to promoting the gimmick that the virus was intentionally leaked from a Chinese laboratory, in order to dilute people's criticism of his incompetence in the pandemic management and governance, while the liberal media have not demonstrated a clearly opposite viewpoint just as they have regarding other issues such as climate change, instead, many have maintained an ambiguous or even congruent attitude. Therefore, liberal media might have also disseminated misinformation and contributed to relevant misperceptions, and this also explains my research findings.

In addition to the main associations, my findings also provided implications regarding how these effects vary across different people. It is intriguing that the effects of both Fox News use and MSNBC use on misperceptions became stronger among those with a liberal ideology. This finding is obviously at odds with most prior research that illustrated the greater effect of conservativism on misperceptions, providing novel evidence of how political ideology affects misperceptions in the context of COVID-19. Findings with regard to the role of NFC was not unexpected though. I found that NFC did not moderate the effect of Fox News use on misperceptions, while the association between MSNBC use and misperceptions was indeed moderated by NFC, that is, among those with a greater preference of cognitive, logical, and statistical information processing, the positive effect of MSNCB use became relatively weaker. Similarly, trust in scientists also moderated the effects of using both partisan media outlets. Specifically, the positive effects were found to become weaker among those with a greater trust in scientists amid the COVID-19 pandemic. When it comes to the role of message derogation, my findings showed that message derogation did mediate the positive ties between using both partisan media and misperceptions. This finding implies that partisan media facilitate and enhance people's misperceptions largely through changing their attitudes toward nonpartisan information and sources. In other words, by providing spun and slanted narratives and depictions, partisan media first foster a derogatory, distrustful attitude of their viewers toward contents on other mass media, then they further lead to people's credulity of misinformation.

2.5 Partisan Media, The Extended Parallel Process Model, and COVID-19 Misperceptions

2.5.1 The Extended Parallel Process Model

As reviewed earlier, partisan media could influence viewers' risk perceptions, affect the extent to which their viewers are confident about their efficacy in navigating through the pandemic, and arouse emotions such as fear. Hence, in this section, I take a step further to include these factors as mediators in the regression models, probing whether there are mediating mechanisms.

Scholars in the field of risk communication have paid tremendous attention to the role of fear appeals (Cho & Salmon, 2006). Among all the theories pertinent to fear appeals, the Extended Parallel Process Model (EPPM hereafter) has been regarded as the most influential in explaining how fear appeals function and proceed (Chen et al., 2021; So, 2013). As a descendant of a series of theories such as the fear-as-acquired drive model (Hovland et al., 1953), the parallel process model (Leventhal, 1970), and the protection motivation theory (Rogers, 1975), the EPPM perfects the integrated process of fear appeals and explicates the reasons that fear appeals fail on some occasions (Witte, 1998a). According to Witte (1992, 1998a), the EPPM suggests that upon exposure to fear-appeal messages, receivers would experience two sequential appraisal processes, respectively. Specifically put, message receivers would initially assess the extent of the threat (i.e., the threat appraisal). Once these people perceive that the threat is not severe enough to make an impact on them, they would not further engage in additional appraisals, ending in no response. Conversely, if the message receivers perceived a high level of threat, they would develop a sense of fear, further motivating them to assuage fear through engaging in the efficacy appraisal. The second appraisal process is, if message receivers perceived that efficacy is greater than threat, then danger control outcome would dominate, evoking behavioral changes in concordance with the recommendations in the message. Otherwise, the receivers would turn to the fear control, leading to defensive avoidance, denial, and reactance (Witte, 1992, 1994; Witte et al., 1996). Since its inception, the EPPM has been extensively examined in a various of contexts, such as meningococcal vaccination (Kuang & Cho, 2016), breast self-examination (Chen & Yang, 2019), and smoking cessation (Chen & Chen, 2021).

Threat, efficacy, and fear are three pivotal constructs in the EPPM (Popova, 2012). Threat can be either a message characteristic or a perceived element. It is fairly common that in experimental studies, messages are intentionally designed to present information about the severity of the threat and the target group's susceptibility to the threat (e.g., Cho & Salmon, 2006). Correspondingly, perceived threat entails perceived severity and perceived susceptibility. The EPPM attaches greater significance to the subjective perception of threat instead of the actual threat (Chen & Yang, 2019). Perceived severity refers to the beliefs in the magnitude of the threat and the seriousness of its consequences. Perceived susceptibility denotes individuals' evaluations on their vulnerability or the possibility that they would experience such threat. For instance, in the context of the COVID-19, the concept of perceived susceptibility is oftentimes operationalized as the extent to which individuals believe that they are at risk of getting infected with the virus (Popova, 2012; Witte, 1998a). When individuals are presented with a fear-appeal message containing the components of threat (i.e., severity and susceptibility), they need to evaluate the threat of the hazard in the first place prior to taking actions further (Witte, 1994). In other words, perceived severity and perceived susceptibility are two fundamental steps in fear-appeal message processing. A moderate-level to a high-level threat perception is required to initiate the emotion of fear, which is associated with the beginning of coping appraisal (Witte, 1992). Therefore, a cognitive process function in a serial manner would emerge; specifically, threat in the message leads to threat perception, and the perceived threat would further prompt fear, which in turn ties to adaptive or maladaptive behaviors. Moreover, the mediating roles of perceived severity and susceptibility are demonstrated by the information utility model (Knobloch-Westerwick et al., 2005), which posits that individuals estimate information utility prior to taking additional information-seeking behaviors. The concept of utility here entails magnitude, likelihood, and immediacy. These dimensions are consistent with the two sub-dimensions of perceived threat in the EPPM (Zhang & Zhou, 2019).

Given the mechanism of the EPPM, it is imperative to analyse the effect of fear in the integrated psychological process. Preceding theories typically take a rational perspective on fear appeal information processing (Zhang & Zhou, 2019). However, the over-emphasis on the cognitive approach and the overlook of the emotional approach have resulted in divergent findings and weak explanatory power (Witte, 1992). In order to fill this gap, Witte (1998a) contends that as an internal emotional reaction, fear can be triggered when a perilous and self-relevant threat is perceived. Fear is a negative emotion characterized by subjective experience (e.g., "I am frightened.") and physiological arousal (e.g., sweating) (Witte, 1994). For one thing, according to the cognitive appraisal theory proposed by Lazarus (1966, 1991), emotional reactions are derived from certain situational factors. Fear is likely to be activated when people feel an immediate, concrete, and overwhelming physical or psychological danger from their surroundings. The conceptualization of danger is akin to that of perceived threat (So, 2013), implying that the cognitive appraisal of the environment-person relationship (i.e., perceived threat) could elicit specific emotions. For another, fear has been regarded as a major predictor of message rejection responses and is not directly hinged on message acceptance outcomes (Witte, 1992, 1994). Nevertheless, some subsequent studies demonstrated that fear arousal could induce health behaviors, such as clicking health risk messages (Zhang & Zhou, 2019), sharing health-related fear-appeal messages on social media (Zhang & Zhou, 2020), motivating people to be involved in argument-based processing and facilitating breast self-examination (Ruiter, Kok,

Verplanken, & Brug, 2001). Despite the inconsistent findings, the mediating role of fear between perceived threat and behavioral intention has been widely supported. Following this vein of research, I include the major factors of the EPPM in the regression models as mediators.

2.5.2 Measurements

In this section, partisan media use is still the independent variable while COVID-19 misperception the dependent variable (COVID-19 misperceptions, [M = 3.47, SD = 1.09, α = 0.95]; Fox News use [M = 3.57, SD = 1.22]; MSNBC news use [M = 3.61, SD = 1.12]), however, I include the five key factors of EPPM to construct a serial mediation model, namely, perceived severity, perceived susceptibility, self-efficacy, and response efficacy. In what follows, I shall detail the ways in which I measure these variables and construct the serial mediation model.

Perceived severity. To evaluate perceived severity, the respondents were required to indicate the extent to which they agree that the COVID-19 pandemic is "severe," "serious," and "significant" (1 = strongly disagree, 5 = strongly agree; M = 3.76, SD = .97, α = .84). This variable essentially investigates how much the respondents think the pandemic is severe.

Perceived susceptibility. To measure perceived susceptibility, the participants were required to indicate the degree to which they agree with the following three statements, "It is likely that I will contract COVID-19," "I am at the risk of getting COVID-19," and "It is possible that I will get COVID-19" (1 = strongly disagree, 5 = strongly agree; M = 4.18, SD = .67, α = .74). In essence, this variable assesses the extent to which the individuals think they are likely to get infected by the COVID-19.

Self-efficacy. To assess self-efficacy, the respondents were asked to indicate the degree to which they agree with the following statements, "I can wear a mask to prevent getting COVID-19," "Vaccination is easy for me to do to prevent COVID-19," and "Social-distancing to prevent COVID-19 is convenient for me" (1 = strongly disagree, 5 = strongly agree; M = 4.23, SD = .67, α = .70). In a nutshell, the measurement of self-efficacy aims at understanding how much the respondents believe that they can cope with the pandemic through applying the recommended measures such as mask-wearing, social distancing, and getting vaccinated.

Response efficacy. To measure response efficacy, the respondents were required to rate the extent to which they agree with the following three statements: "Wearing masks works in preventing COVID-19," "Social distancing is effective in preventing COVID-19," and "If I get vaccinated, I would be less likely to get COVID-19" (1 = strongly disagree, 5 = strongly agree; M = 4.19, SD = .70, α = .72). In other words, this variable examines how much the respondents believe that these recommended measures are effective in preventing the pandemic.

Fear. To assess fear, I asked the respondents to rate the extent to which they felt "fear," "anxious," and "scared" by the information regarding COVID-19 from mass media (1 = none of this feeling, 5 = a great deal of this feeling; M = 2.37, SD = .85, α = .85).

Control variables. Akin to the above section, I also added control variables into the models to remove the concern of spurious effects. The controls included age (M = 37.47, SD = 11.07), gender (44% female, 56% male), race (79.5% White, 20.5% non-whites), education (*Median* = 5 [Bachelor's degree], SD = 0.83), monthly income (*Median* = 4 [$8000-$10,000], SD = 1.61), Party ID (1 = strong Republican, 5 = strong Democrat; M = 3.29, SD = 1.53), interest in news (M = 3.90, SD = 1.06), and interest in politics (M = 3.71, SD = 1.07).

2.5.3 Analytical Strategy

Hayes' (2018) PROCESS macro models 4 and 6 were applied to analyze the model. PROCESS macro model 4 can demonstrate both the main direct effect and the mediation effects, model 6 can exhibit the serial mediation models. In specific, it is proposed that the main direct effects of partisan media use on COVID-19 misperceptions can be mediated by self-efficacy and response efficacy; and there can also be two serial mediation models, namely, the main direct effects of partisan media use on misperceptions can (1) be serially mediated through perceived susceptibility and fear and (2) be serially mediated through perceived severity and fear. In what follows, I shall detail the findings.

2.5.4 Results

According to the PROCESS macro model 6, findings showed that Fox News use was not serially mediated through perceived susceptibility and fear (*Serial mediation effect* = −0.0001, *Boot SE* = 0.0004, 95% CI: [−0.0010, 0.0007]). Approximately 57% of the variance in COVID-19 misperceptions was accounted for by the predictors (R^2 = .57). Specifically, Fox News use was not associated with perceived susceptibility (b = 0.0276, SE = 0.0192, t = 1.4366, p = 0.1512, 95% CI: [−0.0101, 0.0654]), and perceived susceptibility was negatively associated with fear of COVID-19 (b = −0.3361, SE = 0.0417, t = −8.0540, p < 0.001, 95% CI: [−0.4180, −0.2542]), while fear of COVID-19 was not significantly associated with COVID-19 misperceptions (b = 0.0061, SE = 0.0307, t = 0.1976, p = 0.8434, 95% CI: [−0.0541, 0.0662]).

When it comes to the role of MSNBC use, findings of the PROCESS macro model 6 suggested that the effect of consuming MSNBC programs on misperceptions regarding COVID-19 was not serially mediated through perceived susceptibility and fear of COVID-19 (*Serial mediation effect* = 0.0024, *Boot SE* = 0.0015, 95% CI: [−0.0001, 0.0056]). Approximately 41% of the variance in COVID-19 misperceptions was accounted for by the predictors (R^2 = .41). Specifically, MSNBC news use was positively associated with perceived susceptibility (b = 0.1273, SE = 0.0210, t = 6.0658, p < 0.001, 95% CI: [0.0861, 0.1684]), implying that the use of MSNBC news can facilitate perceived susceptibility of COVID-19. Further, perceived susceptibility was negatively associated with fear of COVID-19 ($b = -0.2929$, $SE = 0.0427$, $t = -6.8644$, $p < 0.001$, 95% CI: [-0.3767, -0.2092]), while fear of COVID-19 was not significantly associated with COVID-19 misperceptions ($b = -0.0634$, $SE = 0.0339$, $t = -1.8715$, $p = 0.0616$, 95% CI: [-0.1299, 0.0031]).

Moreover, the findings of the PROCESS macro model 6 indicated that the main effect of Fox News use on COVID-19 misperceptions was not serially mediated through perceived severity and fear of COVID-19 (*Serial mediation effect* $= -0.0011$, *Boot SE* $= 0.0007$, 95% CI: [-0.0028, 0.0000]). Approximately 62% of the variance in COVID-19 misperceptions was accounted for by the predictors ($R^2 = .62$). Specifically, the effect of Fox News use on perceived severity was significant and positive ($b = 0.610$, $SE = 0.0270$, $t = 2.2591$, $p < 0.05$, 95% CI: [0.0080, 0.1140]), implying that the use of Fox News can intensify individuals' perceived severity of the COVID-19 pandemic. Further, perceived severity was negatively associated with fear of COVID-19 ($b = -0.1904$, $SE = 0.0300$, $t = -6.3396$, $p < 0.001$, 95% CI: [-0.2493, -0.1315]), and fear of COVID-19 was in turn positively associated with COVID-19 misperceptions ($b = 0.0986$, $SE = 0.0285$, $t = 3.4538$, $p < 0.001$, 95% CI: [0.0426, 0.1546]).

Furthermore, the findings of the PROCESS macro model 6 suggested that the main effect of MSNBC use on COVID-19 misperceptions was not serially mediated through perceived severity and fear of COVID-19 (*Serial mediation effect* $= -0.0007$, *Boot SE* $= 0.0008$, 95% CI: [-0.0024, 0.0008]). Approximately 47% of the variance in COVID-19 misperceptions was accounted for by the predictors ($R^2 = .47$). Specifically, the effect of MSNBC use on perceived severity was significant and positive ($b = 0.1693$, $SE = 0.0291$, $t = 5.8141$, $p < 0.001$, 95% CI: [0.1121, 0.2264]), implying that the use of MSNBC can intensify individuals' perceived severity of the COVID-19 pandemic. Further, perceived severity was negatively associated with fear of COVID-19 ($b = -0.1436$, $SE = 0.0310$, $t = -4.6270$, $p < 0.001$, 95% CI: [-0.2045, -0.0827]), and fear of COVID-19 was not significantly associated with COVID-19 misperceptions ($b = 0.0283$, $SE = 0.0313$, $t = 0.9046$, $p = 0.3659$, 95% CI: [-0.0331, 0.0897]).

Next, I performed the PROCESS macro model 4 to examine the indirect effect of partisan media use on COVID-19 misperceptions mediated through self-efficacy and response efficacy. First, findings exhibited that self-efficacy significantly mediated the main effect of Fox News use on COVID-19 misperceptions (*Mediation effect* $= -0.0167$, *Boot SE* $= 0.0065$, 95% CI: [-0.0312, -0.0058]). Approximately 57% of the variance in COVID-19 misperceptions was accounted for by the predictors ($R^2 = .57$). Specifically, Fox News use was positively associated with self-efficacy of COVID-19 ($b = 0.0958$, $SE = 0.0191$, $t = 5.0037$, $p < 0.001$, 95% CI: [0.0582, 0.1334]), implying that the use of Fox News can facilitate individuals' perceived self-efficacy. Further, self-efficacy was negatively associated with COVID-19 misperceptions ($b = -0.1740$, $SE = 0.0383$, $t = -4.5447$, $p < 0.001$, 95% CI: [-0.2491, -0.0989]).

Similarly, PROCESS macro model 4 was conducted to explore whether the effect of MSNBC use on COVID-19 misperceptions can also be mediated by self-efficacy. According to the results, there is a significant mediation effect (*Mediation effect* = −0.0201, *Boot SE* = 0.0085, 95% CI: [−0.0380, −0.0041]). Approximately 40% of the variance in COVID-19 misperceptions was accounted for by the predictors (R^2 = .40). Specifically, MSNBC news use was positively associated with self-efficacy of COVID-19 (b = 0.1557, *SE* = 0.0212, t = 7.3582, p < 0.001, 95% CI: [0.1142, 0.1972]), implying that the use of MSNBC news increased people's beliefs that they can apply the recommended measures to cope with the pandemic. Further, self-efficacy in this mediation model was negatively associated with COVID-19 misperceptions (b = −0.1291, *SE* = 0.0425, t = −3.0382, p < 0.01, 95% CI: [−0.2126, −0.0457]).

Akin to the above analyses, PROCESS macro model 4 was also applied to test the mediating role of response efficacy. Specifically, the model illustrated that the response efficacy significantly mediated the main effects of Fox News use on COVID-19 misperceptions (*Mediation effect* = −0.0124, *Boot SE* = 0.0062, 95% CI: [−0.0259, −0.0023]). Approximately 58% of the variance in COVID-19 misperceptions was accounted for by the predictors (R^2 = .58). Specifically, Fox News use was positively associated with response efficacy of COVID-19 (b = 0.0566, *SE* = 0.0202, t = 2.8060, p < 0.01, 95% CI: [0.0170, 0.0961]), implying that the use of Fox News can facilitate people's response efficacy. Further, response efficacy was negatively associated with COVID-19 misperceptions (b = −0.2187, *SE* = 0.0358, t = −6.1140, p < 0.001, 95% CI: [−0.2889, −0.1485]).

Finally, findings again revealed a significant mediation model wherein the association between MSNBC use and COVID-19 misperceptions was mediated by response efficacy (*Mediation effect* = −0.0284, *Boot SE* = 0.0089, 95% CI: [−0.0478, −0.0126]). Approximately 41% of the variance in COVID-19 misperceptions was accounted for by the predictors (R^2 = .41). Specifically, MSNBC use was positively associated with response efficacy of COVID-19 (b = 0.1346, *SE* = 0.0220, t = 6.1074, p < 0.01, 95% CI: [0.0914, 0.1779]), implying that the use of MSNBC programs can also trigger greater response efficacy. Further, response efficacy was negatively associated with COVID-19 misperceptions (b = −0.2106, *SE* = 0.0398, t = −5.2889, p < 0.001, 95% CI: [−0.2887, −0.1324]).

Table 2.3. Direct and indirect effects of partisan media use on COVID-19 misperceptions.

2.5.5 Conclusion and Discussion

Consuming partisan media, shapes individuals' misperceptions not only through eliciting their derogatory attitude toward non-partisan mass media but also through affecting their risk perceptions with respect to the pandemic. The EPPM is the very theory that describes how exposure to information and messages leads to varied extents of risk perceptions and fear. Although the

Table 2.3 Direct and indirect effects of partisan media use on COVID-19 misperceptions

Direct and indirect paths	B (SE)
Independent variable 1: Fox News use	
Fox News use → fear	−0.020(0.024)
Fox News use → perceived susceptibility	0.028(0.019)
Fox News use → perceived susceptibility → COVID-19 misperceptions	−0.143(0.040) ***
Fox News use → perceived susceptibility → fear → COVID-19 misperceptions	0.006(0.031)
Fox News use → perceived severity	0.061(0.027) *
Fox News use → perceived severity → COVID-19 misperceptions	0.281(0.026) ***
Fox News use → perceived severity → fear → COVID-19 misperceptions	0.99(0.29) ***
Fox News use → self-efficacy	0.096(0.019) ***
Fox News use → self-efficacy → COVID-19 misperceptions	−0.174(0.038) ***
Fox News use → response efficacy	0.057(0.020) **
Fox News use → response efficacy → COVID-19 misperceptions	−0.219(0.036) ***
Independent variable 2: MSNBC use	
MSNBC use → fear	−0.059(0.027) *
MSNBC use → perceived susceptibility	0.127(0.210) ***
MSNBC use → perceived susceptibility → COVID-19 misperceptions	−0.293(0.043) ***
MSNBC use → perceived susceptibility → fear → COVID-19 misperceptions	−0.063(0.034)
MSNBC use → perceived severity	0.169(0.029) ***
MSNBC use → perceived severity → COVID-19 misperceptions	0.332(0.029) ***
MSNBC use → perceived severity → fear → COVID-19 misperceptions	0.028(0.031)
MSNBC use → self-efficacy	0.156(0.021) ***
MSNBC use → self-efficacy → COVID-19 misperceptions	−0.129(0.043) **
MSNBC use → response efficacy	0.135(0.22) ***
MSNBC use → response efficacy → COVID-19 misperceptions	−0.211(0.040) ***

Note: Standardized path coefficients were reported with standard errors in parentheses. *$p < .05$, **$p < .01$, ***$p < .001$.

bulk of EPPM studies have been performed through experimentations, such research design could only capture the direct and immediate impacts of experimental stimuli on respondents. Therefore, in this section, I still conduct a traditional survey study to investigate whether the main EPPM constructs, namely, perceived severity, perceived susceptibility, response efficacy, self-efficacy, and fear, could constitute a serial mediation mechanism to influence the main effects of partisan media use on COVID-19 misperceptions. Some intriguing aspects of the findings merits further discussions and explications.

My findings exhibit that using Fox News was not significantly tied to perceived susceptibility whereas utilization of MSNBC was positively associated with perceived susceptibility. The rationale is rather straightforward. A rich body of research guided by the conventional EPPM has shown that, in various contexts, conservative media are more likely to tone down the severity of the risks per se, compared to their liberal counterparts. For instance, a content analysis regarding the newspaper coverage of global warming illustrated that the conservative publication, *The Wall Street Journal*, was least likely to cover the threat posed by global warming among other outlets they analyzed (Feldman et al., 2017). Akin to these studies, research in the context of the COVID-19 pandemic also exhibited that heavy viewers of conservative media sources were not prone to have a greater risk perception than their liberal counterparts (e.g., Borah et al., 2022; Chung & Jones-Jang, 2022; Calvillo et al., 2020; Zhou et al., 2022). The reasons are rather straightforward. In the United States, conservative media reported mounting conspiracy theories and various misleading stories about COVID-19 such as injecting disinfectants could cure the virus (Borah et al., 2022; Rovetta & Bhagavathula, 2020) and taking Vitamin C could prevent infection (Ingraham, 2020; Jamieson & Albarracine, 2020). These unsubstantiated claims would cause a series of adverse effects on the governance of the epidemic, including lowering people's estimates of the cost of epidemic prevention, increasing people's acceptance of conspiracy theories, weakening the credibility of the discourses of the scientific community, depriving people of a guidance worthwhile following, and enable particular agents with special political agendas to spread misinformation and capture personal interests.

Moreover, response efficacy and self-efficacy are also major constructs in the EPPM. Findings showed that viewing Fox News and MSNBC programs can both boost the two types of efficacies. To some extent, this result may be surprising, especially in terms of the positive relationship between Fox News use and both efficacies, but such a positive tie is not without reasons. First, self-efficacy mainly denotes individuals' perception of their own abilities to take measures and cope with the situation. Although Fox News use contributed to misperceptions, it does not influence the extent to which people are confident in their subjective initiative and practical power of action. In other words, although people fall for misinformation and cannot navigate the pandemic with a scientific attitude, they can still hold the belief that it is easy for them to do what experts recommended, and whether they are willing to really abide by those recommendations is another matter. When it comes to response efficacy, Fox News use also had a positive relationship with it. Heavy Fox News viewers are not necessarily outright denying the effectiveness of preventive measures such as vaccinations, mask wearing and social distancing, but they still may not follow these recommendations as their behavior patterns may largely depend on their political stance and even their religious beliefs. For example, an ultra-conservative U.S. citizen might engage in self-identity construction and ideological exhibition through vocally expressing derogation and disdain for the recommended measures. In this case, it no longer matters how high their response efficacy is.

2.6 Incidental News Exposure and COVID-19 Misperceptions

2.6.1 Incidental News Exposure

A great deal of theories in communication studies underscore the role of active attention to news in affecting perception shaping, knowledge acquisition, and some behavioural outcomes (e.g., Hardy & Scheufele, 2005; Shah et al., 2007; Yamamoto & Nah, 2018). For instance, the Cognitive Mediation Model (CMM hereafter) describes a serially mediating path wherein individuals' proactive surveillance of news and attention to news could elicit cognitive elaboration, which in turn leads to learning (Eveland Jr., 2001; Eveland Jr. et al., 2003). Communication mediation model describes that the association between people's orientations and political engagement is mediated by communication patterns, such as hard news media use and political discussions (Gil de Zúñiga et al., 2019; McLeod et al., 1994; Sotirovic & McLeod, 2001). However, these media effects theories have two transparent limitations, first, they focus primarily on the possible outcomes of audiences actively paying attention to the news, rather than whether people's incidental exposure to information also have similarly strong media effects. Second, these theories were mainly developed in the era when traditional mass media prevailed, hence, their explanatory power should be questioned in the current social media age when the relationship between consumers and content providers have already been fundamentally revolutionized (Tewksbury et al., 2001). In light of these gaps and limitations, this section examines the extent to which incidentally exposing to news on traditional media could affect misperceptions regarding COVID-19. In other words, incidental news exposure serves as the independent variable in this section.

The previous section mainly details the impact of proactive use of partisan media on people's misperceptions regarding COVID-19, positing that learning and perception formation are essentially active processes in which people might be motivated to seek out and retain information about issues of interest. However, not all knowledge obtained from media comes from active seeking and learning. Even those with limited interest in specific issues can still learn from media, in this case, knowledge acquisition and subsequent perception forming are not hinged on active learning, instead, it relies on passive learning. As its name suggests, passive learning typically occurs "in the absence of a motivation to become informed" (Tewksbury et al., 2001, p. 534). In other words, passive learning describes the situation that individuals acquire certain knowledge or get informed in an accidental way without actively seeking for relevant information out of their needs or being motivated by certain political ideology. Therefore, such information gain requires a minimal level of attention to the media.

In the context of the COVID-19 pandemic, information gain through an incidental style is all too common. As a one-in-a-century major global health crisis, the COVID-19 pandemic has already led to information overload and explosion, making it almost impossible for people to avoid relevant information as long as they live in this modern society. Although information avoidance and information detox might assist people to temporarily escape from the state of information overload and even information fatigue to a certain extent, this strategy cannot absolutely isolate people from the entire information environment. After all, ambient news has become ubiquitous, and online and offline information have also become fully intertwined.

In fact, incidental news exposure (INE) is not a brand-new concept, while it has always been an important idea in the media effect research (Karnowski et al., 2017; Kim et al., 2013; Strauß et al., 2020; Tewksbury et al., 2001). Downs (1957) has conceptualized accidental information exposure as "accruing to [information] without any special effort on his part to find" (p.233). In essence, INE describes citizens encountering news in an accidental way or just through serendipitous inadvertent exposure; altering their media practices (Boczkowski et al., 2018), and influencing their political knowledge or knowledge about public affairs (Kim et al., 2013). Upon decades of academic discussions and debates, the conceptualization of INE has become much more multidimensional and abundant. For example, Rubin (1984) identified two prominent motivations of media use, namely, instrumental motivation and ritual motivation. Instrumentally motivated media use indicates purposive consumption, whilst ritually motivated media use pertains to the less active information exposure (Kim et al., 2013; Rubin, 1984). In addition, Wieland and Kleinen-von Königslöw (2020) conceptualized a triple-path model of INE on social media as a process, namely, automatic, incidental, and active pathways. Hence, in a nutshell, INE highlights the unintentionality of news exposure (Fletcher & Nielsen, 2018; Kaiser et al., 2021; Tewksbury et al., 2001; Yamamoto & Morey, 2019). Many subsequent studies have developed several theoretical models to enrich the conceptualization of INE. For example, in the realm of political communication studies, Matthes and associates (2020) have formulated a Political Incidental Exposure News (PINE) Model. The PINE Model basically splits the original concept of INE into two dimensions, namely, the passive overview of "incidentally encountered political information" and the active processing of "incidentally encountered content appraised as relevant" (Matthes et al., 2020, p. 1031).

Against this backdrop, INE has become increasingly important to ensure that "citizens encounter counter-attitudinal information or at least remain connected to the political public sphere" (Goyanes & Demeter, 2022, p. 78). A large proportion of INE research has been dedicated to the investigations of its antecedents, consequences, and classifications. In terms of the antecedents of INE, previous studies indicated that INE usually occurs when individuals' networks are able to provide enough content to fulfil their needs; if not, they would otherwise seek out for information more purposefully. News consumers' news preferences, uses and trust also affect their probability to be incidentally exposed to news (Goyanes, 2020).

When it comes to the consequences of INE, a series of scholars, through empirical investigations, have identified that compared to active news seeking, INE could also lead to online and offline political participation (Kim et al., 2013; Valeriani & Vaccari, 2016), cognitive elaboration, and thorough information engagement such as thoroughly following through the entire news piece upon accidental exposure to a headline, clicking on the news link and listening or reading the entire news piece, as well as reading the entire news article until the end (Chen et al., 2022; Gil de Zúñiga et al., 2021; Heiss & Matthes, 2021; Shahin et al., 2021; Wieland & Kleinen-von Königslöw, 2020). It is safe to say that even if people get exposed to news in an incidental way, certain triggers in the information such as unexpected, attractive, or surprising elements can still direct people to further elaborate on the news more consciously and effortfully afterwards. Furthermore, the extant literature has exhibited pluralistic evidence of the effects of INE on knowledge acquisition. More specifically, many studies found that INE is not a significant predictor of learning, or that the influence of INE on learning is conditional and indirect (e.g., Gil de Zúñiga et al., 2021), whereas some demonstrated that INE can straightforwardly effectively facilitate knowledge acquisition among citizens (Anderson et al., 2021; Nanz & Matthes, 2020; Shehata et al., 2015; Takano et al., 2021). Feezell (2018) even found that INE on social media could exert an agenda-setting effect, especially on the low political interest public.

Plenty of INE research have classified the concept according to the specific outlets through which people get exposed to information incidentally. With the rise of social media platforms, recent INE research mainly focuses on the role of social media INE in shaping perceptions, attitudes, and behaviors (e.g., Ahmed & Gil-Lopez, 2022; Schäfer, 2023; Strauß et al., 2020). Besides, a handful of studies have also endeavored to examine whether INE to traditional media contents could exert a significant impact on its viewers (Baum, 2002, Downs, 1957; Tewksbury et al., 2001). In this section, I first investigate the relationship between traditional INE and COVID-19 misperceptions. Prior research in the similar vein has demonstrated that social media INE could intensify people's general misperceptions and COVID-19-specific misperceptions because of the missing of the institutional gatekeeper on social media platforms, enabling not only incidental authentic information exposure but also incidental misinformation exposure (Borah et al., 2022). If the positive tie between social media INE and misperceptions is hinged upon the special characteristics of the information dissemination mechanism of social media platforms, then INE to traditional media may not necessarily contribute to misperceptions. However, this remains an open question because to the best of my knowledge, the extant literature has not yet rendered sufficient evidence regarding the extent to which traditional media INE is tied to misperceptions. Considering this gap, I investigate the effects of INE to three typical traditional media, TV, newspapers, and radios, on COVID-19 misperceptions.

2.6.2 Media Locus of Control

Akin to the previous section, I argue that the effects of INE, if any, on misperceptions do not occur equally amongst all people. This idea is also in line with the development directionality of a bulk of political communication theories such as the communication mediation model, that is, to explore more nuanced media effects by incorporating more mediating and moderating factors. In this section, I include media locus of control as a moderator to explore whether the impacts of INE to the three different outlets differ across people with varying levels of media locus of control.

Media locus of control (MLOC) is defined as "the extent to which an individual believes they control media influences" (Maksl et al., 2015, p. 33). In terms of its operationalization, MLOC is typically measured by asking respondents to indicate the extent to which they agree with several statements, including that if they were misled by misinformation and disinformation on news media, it is their own behaviors that determines how soon they would learn credible information; they are in control of the information they could obtain from the news media; and that when they were misinformed by the news media, they themselves were to blame (Borah, 2022). The idea of MLOC was originated from the concept of locus of control (LOC), which refers to the "mastery of one's environment" (p. 162) and people's belief that their behaviors are under their own control (Rubin, 1993). In essence, people with a greater level of LOC typically hold that their own life experiences are the outcomes of their own choices and behaviors, instead of their fate, luck, or external factors such as influential others or the environment (Koo, 2009).

Given its conceptualization, MLOC's being incorporated as a moderator is justified. As I reviewed earlier, INE refers to accidental exposure to information. This concept obviously does not focus on whether people have a strong locus of control over their media environment, and because of this, people typically do not practice consumptive news feed curation. Therefore, misinformation is likely to sneak in when people do not take the initiative to control and curate their own media environment, contributing to the likely positive association between INE and misperceptions. But in any case, this is merely a speculation, and it is not yet clear whether the relationship between INE and misperception varies with the degree of media locus of control. Therefore, I take a step further to use MLOC as a moderator, evaluating its role in differing the main effects of INE to TV, newspapers, and radios on COVID-19 misperceptions.

2.6.3 Discussion Network Heterogeneity

Political discussion is deemed the hallmark of a functioning democracy because it is typically motivated by two defining characteristics, namely, opinion forming and persuasion (Gil de Zúñiga et al., 2016; McLeod et al., 1994). Frequent and healthy political discussion can facilitate free flow of information, which is conducive for the free marketplace of opinions and satisfies the essential demands of deliberative democracy (Gil de Zúñiga et al., 2016; Su & Xiao, 2022). A central component of political discussion is expression. Expression is considered quite psychologically demanding and mentally clarifying, namely, it witnesses the transformation of private thoughts into publicly available ones, hence, discursive communication and interpersonal political discussion can promote political thinking and political participation. For instance, political discussion can advance the changing and development of the discussed topics, thereby stimulating continuous thinking and further persuading or responding to the communication partners (Shah, 2016). In some transitional democracies, the role of political discussion is more important because it not only serves as the purpose of communication but "is also considered a small piece woven in a broader social fabric—civic cultures" (Su & Xiao, 2022, p. 211). Namely, political discussion reinforces "the parameters and impact of civic cultures on political situations" (Dahlgren, 2005, p. 159).

A large number of political communication theories have emphasized the irreplaceably important role of political discussion, especially its influence in promoting political participation. One representative theoretical framework is the differential gains model, which aptly highlights that hard news media use has an overall positive effect on political participation, while such main effect is contingent upon the frequency with which people talk to others about political issues (Scheufele, 2002). More specifically, among those who frequently involve in political discussions, the effect of hard news media use on political participation is stronger compared to those not frequently engage in political discussions (Hardy & Scheufele, 2005; Su & Xiao, 2022).

The significance of political discussion has become a truism in decades of research on media effects and political participation. In these studies, political discussion is typically measured by the frequency with which people engage in interpersonal discussions about political matters or public affairs. However, in addition to the frequency of discussion, the extent to which people's discussion network is heterogeneous has become another research focus. Discussion network heterogeneity refers to how likely and how frequently people talk about public affairs with others of oppositional viewpoints or of different socioeconomic statuses, gender groups, and age groups (e.g., Kim et al., 2013; Lee et al., 2014; Scheufele et al., 2006). People encountering diverse and pluralistic opinions and engaging in heterogeneous discussion networks are easily forced to "compromise between different viewpoints" (Scheufele et al., 2006, p. 730), thus being motivated to search for further knowledges and develop better understanding to complex issues (Scheufele et al., 2006; Kim et al., 2013).

By its conceptualization, it can be easily inferred that discussion network heterogeneity could alleviate or even resolve the adverse ramifications of echo chamber. It has been comprehensively agreed that the echo chambers can make people no longer focus on the evidence and details that possibly buttress the facts, while paying more attention to the emotional expression that could support their own pre-existing ideas, beliefs, and values. The popularity of weak ties and the richness of technological affordances on social media platforms also make it easy for people to stay in the echo chambers and keep resonating with those sharing homogeneous views, thus avoiding potential conflicts and confrontations. On the surface, this shows an empowerment for users to customize their personal news feeds and networks. However, in the long run, this phenomenon will obviously make the misinformation beliefs more solidified and harder to correct, and it will also intensify the affective polarizations among heterogeneous groups, which is unfavorable to the healthy information flow. Clearly, what we call the political discussions that is the bedrock of a democratic society does not include the kind of discussions that only occur in homogeneous networks (Cinelli et al., 2021; Törnberg, 2022).

In this section, I examine whether discussion network heterogeneity can also play a moderating role to condition the main effects of traditional media INE on COVID-19 misperceptions. I deem this attempt imperative because a heterogeneous network can contribute positively to learning (Bode & Vraga, 2018; Jost et al., 2018; Röchert et al., 2022; Zollo & Quattrociocchi, 2018). For instance, in the context of COVID-19, people discussing conspiracist ideas oftentimes face the risk of being caught in echo chambers, which are oftentimes hyper homogeneous discussion networks. In this case, only through engaging in heterogeneous discussion networks and exposing oneself to oppositional ideas and viewpoints, can self- and social corrections be possible (Bode & Vraga, 2018; Su, 2021). The idea that I include discussion network heterogeneity here as a moderator is that I would like to examine whether COVID-19 misperceptions would be weakened among those who are in a highly heterogeneous discussions and prefer encountering diversified ideas. Previous studies have already lent some empirical evidence showing that discussion network heterogeneity moderated certain media effects. For instance, Su et al. (2022) suggested that the influence of partisan media utilization on COVID-19 misperceptions was weaker among those of a more heterogeneous discussion network. Likewise, Zhang (2023) illustrated that among people with a more heterogeneous network, the effect of information repertoire filtration on social media political expression was stronger. Along this line of thought, we can be confident that the discussion network heterogeneity plays a positive role in assisting people to avoid the various dire consequences of echo chambers.

2.6.4 *Defensive Avoidance*

As I have mentioned in previous sections, approaches of fear control are two-fold, namely, news derogation and defensive avoidance (Roberto et al., 2021; Stephenson & Witte, 1998). In the above section I showcased that partisan media shape their viewers' misperceptions through enhancing and solidifying their derogatory attitudes toward non-partisan, mass media contents in the first place. In other words, to promote misperceptions among its viewers, the very first step was to convince them that contents provided by outlets other than themselves are unreliable. In this section, I attempt to examine whether another fear-control approach, defensive avoidance, could also play a significant mediating role.

Defensive avoidance involves conscious efforts in avoiding specific messages or scenarios, such as leaving a specific webpage, ignoring a dialogue, or changing the channel to prevent exposure to some specific information

(Kessels et al., 2014; McMahan et al., 1998). In fact, in some experimental conditions, utilization of fear-arousing messages is not without reasons. Typically, experimentalists attempt to arouse their respondents' emotion of fear to encourage and motivate them to involve in health promoting and disease-preventive behaviors (Kessels et al., 2014). For instance, to encourage people to quit smoking, experimenters typically include some fear-appeal elements in their experimental materials, such as morbid images of smokers, which might elicit people's defensive avoidance or message derogation. These types of experiments are usually committed to improve health persuasion strategies. More specifically, if fear-appeal messages in experimental stimuli were found to significantly trigger respondents' avoidance behavior or derogatory attitude, such messages would be regarded as effective and will in turn be used in tobacco control advertisements or relevant health campaigns. In the context of partisan media effects, we can infer that heavy partisan media users might be more prone to develop a reliance on partisan heuristic cues and thus instinctively avoid contents at odds they the cues they are accustomed to. This behavior might be out of an instinctive evasion of cognitive dissonance, and it is also a manifestation of confirmation bias. For instance, long term Fox News users might have already been quite familiar with the discourses such as that climate change is a hoax. When they encounter information incongruent with these partisan heuristic cues or frames, they may be unwilling to accept the challenge of their belief system that such heterogeneous information poses. At this moment, defensive avoidance will appear (Dalege & van der Does, 2022; Gilad et al., 1987).

Although defensive avoidance is oftentimes examined in experimental scenarios with specific message stimuli provided to respondents, it also possibly occurs in non-experimental situations just as message derogation does. Unfortunately, the extant literature does not show sufficient evidence regarding the association between INE and defensive avoidance. In this section, I am interested in whether people would defensively avoid information upon incidentally exposing them from TV, newspapers, and radio. Although the relevant literature is far from sufficient, I infer that there may be a positive tie between the INE and defensive avoidance, because the occurrence of INE is not premised on people's active information seeking, that is to say, information that comes across accidentally is likely to have nothing to do with people's initial interests, nor does it satisfy people's information needs. Therefore, people may actively avoid as they are not interested or do not want unexpected information to disturb their current situation.

In the analysis, I incorporate defensive avoidance as a mediating variable, namely, I explore whether INE to the three types of traditional media would first lead to viewers' defensive avoidance of COVID-19 related information mass media, which in turn contributes to increased misperceptions. Prior studies have already lent rich evidence to support how defensive avoidance could mediate media effects on perception forming and behavioral change. For instance, Goodall and Reed (2013) suggested that as a type of maladaptive responses to fear appeal messages, defensive avoidance occurs when individuals are exposed to stories referencing uncertainty regarding feasibility or effectiveness of proposed solutions. McKay et al. (2004) revealed that when their experimental respondents were exposed to messages containing low level of efficacy, they were prone to defensively avoid such messages. Roberto et al. (2021) also found that perceived threat and perceived efficacy discouraged maladaptive fear control responses such as defensive avoidance prior to stimulating behavioral responses. Through mediation analysis, I attempt to investigate whether INE to the three traditional types of media would lead people to avoid COVID-19 information, which in turn affect misperceptions.

2.6.5 *Measurements*

In this section, I use two survey data collected from the U.S. and China, respectively, to exhibit a cross-national comparison. However, due to the way the questionnaire is designed, and the different variables utilized in both samples, I only use the variable defensive avoidance to construct a mediation model when studying the U.S. sample. Moreover, I use COVID-19 factual knowledge as the dependent variable in the Chinese sample, rather than COVID-19 misperceptions. The main reason was that several items used to measure misperceptions in the U.S. sample involved conspiracy theories related to China, such as the claim that the virus was intentionally created and leaked from Chinese lab. These items are obviously inapplicable in the Chinese questionnaire. With this in mind, in my interpretation of the survey results in China, if INE is found to negatively correlate with COVID-19 factual knowledge level, then it can be considered that INE actually leads to misperceptions, or at least a reduction in COVID-19 factual knowledge level. After all, in terms of their operationalizations, knowledge level and misperceptions are contradictory concepts.

In addition to this mediating variable and the dependent variable, the independent variables and the two moderating variables are the same in both samples. Therefore, taken together, in the U.S. sample, I explore (1) the main effects of INE to three traditional types of media on COVID-19 misperceptions, (2) the moderating effects of MLOC and discussion network heterogeneity on the three main effects, respectively, and (3) the mediating effect of defensive avoidance on the three main effects. In the Chinese sample, I investigate (1) the main effects of INE to three traditional types of media on COVID-19 knowledge level and (2) the moderating effects of MLOC and discussion network heterogeneity on the three main associations, respectively.

The U.S. data used for analysis in this section is the same set with that of the previous two sections. Specifically, the fieldwork of the U.S. survey was performed in October 2021. I recruited survey respondents through Amazon MTurk. The respondents of this survey were individuals that resided in the U.S. at the time the questionnaire was completed, and only those above the age of 18 were recruited in this sampling. Each respondent was compensated with 1.1 dollar. As a result, 1004 individuals took part in the survey. Upon collection of the initial data, I removed incomplete sample, which yielded 915 samples as final valid samples.

As for the Chinese sample, I performed an online survey between November 1st and 15th, 2022, and all participants were recruited through a Chinese crowdsourcing company extensively utilized for survey sampling, *Wenjuanxing*. The initial raw data comprises 1,465 respondents aged 18 or above who resided in the mainland China. Each respondent was compensated with 15 Chinese Yuan, which is approximately equivalent to US$2.18 based on the exchange rate at the time of data collection. Upon raw data collection, data cleaning was proceeded in two steps. In the first step, all the incomplete samples were removed. Next, the crowdsourcing company's website was able to identify the time duration each participant spent on completing the questionnaire. According to Amazeen (2020), samples that spent less than the median time to complete the questionnaire are considered speeders, who might have provided low-quality data. Hence, I further removed samples that spent 18 or fewer minutes (*Median* = 36 mins). Finally, I yielded 1333 valid samples for analysis.

INE to TV. INE to TV was measured by a single item asking about the frequencies with which the respondents "unintentionally encounter news from TV" via a 5-point Likert scale (1 = never, 5 = always; $M_{U.S.}$ = 3.80, $SD_{U.S.}$ = 1.10; M_{China} = 3.30, SD_{China} = 1.02).

INE to newspapers. INE to newspapers was measured by a single item asking about the frequencies with which the respondents "unintentionally encounter news from newspapers" via a 5-point Likert scale (1 = never, 5 = always; $M_{U.S.}$ = 3.64, $SD_{U.S.}$ = 1.28; M_{China} = 2.28, SD_{China} = 1.12).

INE to radios. INE to radios was measured by a single item asking about the frequencies with which the respondents "unintentionally encounter news from radios" via a 5-point Likert scale (1 = never, 5 = always; $M_{U.S.}$ = 3.42, $SD_{U.S.}$ = 1.14; M_{China} = 2.75, SD_{China} = 1.15).

COVID-19 misperceptions (the U.S. sample). The measurement of the COVID-19 misperceptions consists of nine items. Each item was a piece of misinformation or conspiracy theory, and the respondents were asked to indicate the extent to which they agree with each statement on a 5-point Likert scale (1 = strongly disagree, 5 = strongly agree). The statements include "COVID-19 death rates are inflated," "Wearing a mask does not protect you from COVID-19," "5G radiant is the real cause of COVID-19," "Bill Gates intends to implant microchips in people via COVID-19 vaccination," and so forth. What needs to be reiterated is that misinformation and conspiracy theories do not necessarily mean that the message is fake, it highlights that the information per se lacks scientific evidence and can facilitate the devastation of the "infodemic" (Himelboim et al., 2023). The measurement of this variable reached satisfactory internal reliability (*M* = 3.47, *SD* = 1.09, α = 0.95).

COVID-19 knowledge level (the Chinese sample). Adapted from prior research (Austin et al., 2021), knowledge about COVID-19 was measured with true-or-false statements, with correct answers totaled, based on information from the World Health Organization (2020), the Centers for Disease Control and Prevention (2020), and a contemporary RTI (2020) survey. Respondents were asked to select true or false for the following seven statements: "Antibiotics can be used to treat the COVID-19 virus." "People of all ages can become infected with the COVID-19." "People of all ethnic groups can become infected with the COVID-19." "Eating garlic can lower your chances of getting infected with the COVID-19 virus." "Most people who are infected with COVID-19 virus die from it." "Most people who are infected with the COVID-19 virus recover from it." And "Older adults or those with compromised immune systems are at a higher risk" ($M = .90$, $SE = .16$, $\alpha = .88$).

Media locus of control. Media locus of control was assessed through three items that asked the respondents to indicate the extent to which they agree with the following three statements, "If I am misled by the rumor on news media, it is my own behavior that determines how soon I will learn credible information," "I am in control of the information I get from the news media," and "When I am misinformed by the news media, I am to blame" ($1 =$ strongly disagree, $5 =$ strongly agree; $M_{U.S.} = 3.98$, $SD_{U.S.} = 0.71$, $\alpha_{U.S.} = 0.74$; $M_{China} = 3.73$, $SD_{China} = .57$; $\alpha_{U.S.} = 0.75$).

Discussion network heterogeneity. Discussion network heterogeneity was assessed by the frequencies with which the respondents "discuss public affairs with the following people," "people who have different viewpoints with you," "people who you disagree with," "people from different race or ethnicity," and "people from different social class" via a 5-point Likert scale ($1 =$ never, $5 =$ always; $M_{U.S.} = 3.60$, $SD_{U.S.} = 0.74$, $\alpha_{U.S.} = 0.76$; $M_{China} = 2.85$, $SD_{China} = 0.72$; $\alpha_{U.S.} = 0.75$).

Defensive avoidance. Defensive avoidance of COVID-19 related topics was measured by the extent to which the respondents agree with the following three statements, "When the topic of COVID-19 comes up in mass media, I'm likely to change the channel," "to avoid reading the coverage," and "to tune it out" ($1 =$ strongly disagree, $5 =$ strongly agree; $M_{U.S.} = 3.57$, $SD_{U.S.} = 1.13$, $\alpha_{U.S.} = 0.89$).

Control variables. Akin to the above sections, I included control variables into the models to remove the concern of spurious effects. The controls included age ($M_{U.S.} = 37.47$, $SD_{U.S.} = 11.07$; $M_{China} = 37.64$, $SD_{China} = 11.29$), gender (U.S.: 44% female, 56% male; China: female: 55.4%, male: 44.6%), race (79.5% White, 20.5% non-whites), education ($Median_{U.S.} = 5$ [Bachelor's degree], $SD_{U.S.} = 0.83$), monthly income ($Median_{U.S.} = 4$ [$8000-$10,000], $SD = 1.61$; $Median_{China} = 3$ [10,0000–30,0000 CNY], $SD_{China} = 1.06$), Party ID ($1 =$ strong Republican, $5 =$ strong Democrat; $M = 3.29$, $SD = 1.53$), interest in news ($M_{U.S.} = 3.90$, $SD_{U.S.} = 1.06$; $M_{China} = 3.92$, $SD_{China} = 0.81$), and interest in politics ($M_{U.S.} = 3.71$, $SD_{U.S.} = 1.07$; $M_{China} = 3.83$, $SD_{China} = 0.64$). It should be noted that race and Party ID were only used as control variables in the U.S. sample because both factors do not apply in China.

2.6.6 Analytical Strategy

To examine the direct effects of INE on COVID-19 misperceptions (U.S.) and factual knowledge of COVID-19 (China), I use hierarchical regression. In terms of the mediation effect of defensive avoidance of COVID-19 news, Hayes' (2018) PROCESS macro model 4 was performed. To investigate the moderating roles of media locus of control and discussion network heterogeneity, I applied Hayes' (2018) PROCESS macro model 1.

2.6.7 Results

I first analyze the U.S. data. As can be seen in Table 2.4, according to the hierarchical regression model, beyond all controls, first, incidental news exposure to TV has positive effects on defensive avoidance of news regarding COVID-19 ($b = 0.200$, $SE = 0.033$, $p < .001$) and COVID-19 misperceptions ($b = 0.201$, $SE = 0.028$, $p < .001$). Moreover, incidental news exposure to newspapers also has positive effects

Table 2.4 Main direct effects of INE on COVID-19 misperceptions.

	Defensive Avoidance			COVID-19 Misperceptions		
Step 1	*B*	*SE*	*t*	*B*	*SE*	*t*
Constant	5.41***	0.28	19.39	4.86***	0.26	18.97
Age	−0.01**	0.003	−3.03	−0.01**	0.003	−2.81
Gender	−0.37***	0.07	−5.52	−0.43***	0.06	−6.92
Race	−0.27***	0.03	−10.49	−0.21***	0.02	−10.79
Education	−0.23***	0.05	−4.82	−0.24***	0.04	−5.45
Monthly income	0.25***	0.02	10.91	0.28***	0.02	13.24
Party ID	−0.08***	0.02	−3.64	−0.11***	0.02	−4.95
News interest	0.01	0.05	0.14	0.11*	0.04	2.56
Political interest	0.01	0.04	0.26	0.03	0.04	0.76
R^2	0.25***			0.31***		
Step 2						
Constant	3.00***	0.28	10.85	2.26***	0.24	9.62
Age	−0.002	0.003	−0.78	−0.001	0.002	−0.03
Gender	−0.19**	0.06	−3.27	−0.23***	0.05	−4.70
Race	−0.16***	0.02	−7.05	−0.14***	0.02	−7.08
Education	−0.16***	0.04	−3.94	−0.17***	0.04	−4.75
Monthly income	0.12***	0.21	5.65	0.14***	0.02	7.57
Party ID	−0.06**	0.02	−2.85	−0.08***	0.02	−4.46
News interest	−0.05	0.04	−1.40	0.04	0.03	1.24
Political interest	−0.05	0.04	−1.21	−0.03	0.03	−0.95
INE to TV	0.20***	0.03	6.02	0.20***	0.03	7.11
INE to newspapers	0.27***	0.03	8.92	0.30***	0.03	11.41
INE to radio	0.12***	0.03	4.21	0.15***	0.02	5.94
R^2	0.45***			0.57***		

Notes: Cell entries (b) are unstandardized betas. SE: Standard error. INE: incidental news exposure. *$p < .05$, **$p < .01$, ***$p < .001$.

on defensive avoidance of news regarding COVID-19 ($b = 0.272$, $SE = 0.031$, $p < .001$) and COVID-19 misperceptions ($b = 0.297$, $SE = 0.026$, $p < .001$). Similarly, incidental news exposure to radios also has positive influences on defensive avoidance of news regarding COVID-19 ($b = 0.121$, $SE = 0.029$, $p < .001$) and COVID-19 misperceptions ($b = 0.145$, $SE = 0.024$, $p < .001$). These findings suggest that the more frequently individuals incidentally exposing themselves to news from TV, newspapers, and radios, the more likely they will defensively avoid COVID-19 related news and fall for misperceptions regarding the pandemic.

Moreover, I am interested in whether there is a mediation effect. Specifically, I strive to understand whether defensive avoidance of COVID-19 news can mediate the associations between INE and misperceptions. Therefore, I conduct Hayes' (2018) PROCESS macro model 4 to investigate the indirect effects. As can be seen in Table 2.5, the model exhibited that defensive avoidance of COVID-19 news significantly mediated the main effects of INE to TV on COVID-19 misperceptions (*Mediation effect* = 0.2409, *Boot SE* = 0.0235, 95% CI: [0.1951, 0.2877]). Approximately 71% of the variance in COVID-19 misperceptions was accounted for by the predictors ($R^2 = .71$). Specifically, INE to TV was positively associated with defensive avoidance of COVID-19 news ($b = 0.3971$, $SE = 0.0293$, $t = 13.5468$, $p < 0.001$, 95% CI: [0.3395, 0.4546]), implying that the incidentally exposing to TV news can intensify people's likelihood of defensive avoidance. Further, defensive avoidance of COVID-19 news positively predicted COVID-19 misperceptions ($b = 0.6066$, $SE = 0.0216$, $t = 28.0412$, $p < 0.001$, 95% CI: [0.5642, 0.6491]).

Furthermore, the indirect effect of INE to newspapers on COVID-19 misperceptions mediated through defensive avoidance is also significant (*Mediation effect* = 0.2353, *Boot SE* = 0.0226, 95% CI: [0.1927, 0.2800]). Approximately 73% of the variance in COVID-19 misperceptions was accounted for by the predictors ($R^2 = .73$). Specifically, INE to newspapers was positively associated with defensive avoidance of COVID-19 news ($b = 0.4106$, $SE = 0.0255$, $t = 16.1103$, $p < 0.001$, 95% CI: [0.3606, 0.4606]), implying that the incidentally exposing to newspaper coverage can also facilitate people's likelihood of defensive avoidance of COVID-19 news, which, in turn, leads to increased COVID-19 misperceptions ($b = 0.5730$, $SE = 0.0219$, $t = 26.1581$, $p < 0.001$, 95% CI: [0.5301, 0.6160]).

Table 2.5 Direct and indirect effects of partisan media use on COVID-19 misperceptions

Indirect paths	B (SE)
INE to TV → defensive avoidance → COVID-19 misperceptions	0.2409(0.0235) ***
INE to newspapers → defensive avoidance → COVID-19 misperceptions	0.2353(0.0226) ***
INE to radios → defensive avoidance → COVID-19 misperceptions	0.1791(0.0236) ***

Note: Standardized path coefficients were reported with standard errors in parentheses. INE: incidental news exposure. *$p < .05$, **$p < .01$, ***$p < .001$.

Finally, findings again reveal a significant indirect effect of INE to radios on COVID-19 misperceptions through defensive avoidance (*Mediation effect* = 0.1791, *Boot SE* = 0.0236, 95% CI: [0.1347, 0.2265]). Approximately 70% of the variance in COVID-19 misperceptions was accounted for by the predictors (R^2 = .70). Specifically, INE to radios positively predicted defensive avoidance of COVID-19 news (*b* = 0.2774, *SE* = 0.0299, *t* = 9.2770, *p* < 0.001, 95% CI: [0.2187, 0.3360]), which indicate that the incidentally exposing to radio programs can also boost individuals' likelihood of defensive avoidance of COVID-19 news, which, in turn, triggered COVID-19 misperceptions (*b* = 0.6456, *SE* = 0.0210, *t* = 30.8106, *p* < 0.001, 95% CI: [0.6045, 0.6867]).

In addition, this section also seeks to unpack conditional effects. Put differently, I assume that the main direct effects of INE to the three media on COVID-19 misperceptions can be varied by individuals' media locus of control and discussion network heterogeneity. To fulfil this goal, Hayes' (2018) PROCESS macro model 1 was performed to investigate the moderation effects.

First, according to the output of PROCESS macro model 1, after controlling for all covariates, the result of the 95% bias-corrected confidence intervals from 5,000 bootstrapped samples demonstrated that the main association between INE to TV and COVID-19 misperceptions was significantly moderated by individuals' media locus of control (*b* = 0.2170, *Boot SE* = 0.0285, *t* = 7.6125, *p* < .001, 95% CI = [0.1611, 0.2730]). Figure 2.6 visualizes the interaction effect. Specifically, among those having greater perceived media locus of control, the effect of INE to TV on COVID-19 misperceptions became stronger

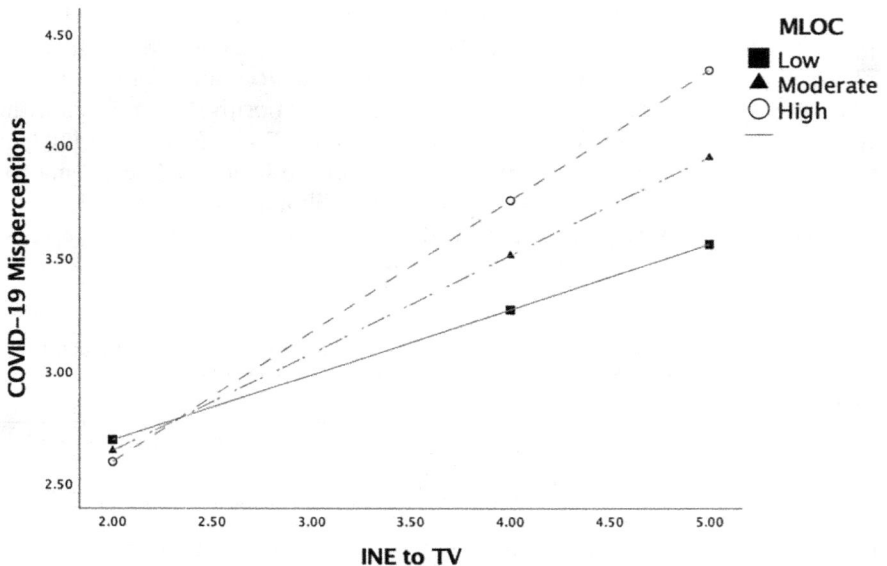

Figure 2.6 Two-way interaction between INE to TV and MLOC on COVID-19 misperceptions (US data).

(*Effect* = 0.5777, *SE* = 0.0347, *t* = 16.6673, *p* < .001, 95% CI = [0.5097, 0.6458]), compared to those with moderate (*Effect* = 0.4330, *SE* = 0.0255, *t* = 17.0059, *p* < .001, 95% CI = [0.3831, 0.4830]) and lower level of media locus of control (*Effect* = 0.2883, *SE* = 0.0286, *t* = 10.0819, *p* < .001, 95% CI = [0.2322, 0.3445]).

Further, the direct effect of INE to newspapers on COVID-19 misperceptions was also significantly moderated by MLOC. Specifically, the 95% bias-corrected confidence intervals from 5,000 bootstrapped samples displayed a significant moderation model (*b* = 0.1874, *SE* = 0.0239, *t* = 7.9230, *p* < .001, 95% CI = [0.1425, 0.2363]). Figure 2.7 showcases the interaction effect. Specifically, among those having greater perceived media locus of control, the effect of INE to newspapers on COVID-19 misperceptions became stronger (*Effect* = 0.5440, *SE* = 0.0261, *t* = 20.8092, *p* < .001, 95% CI = [0.4927, 0.5953]), compared to those with moderate (*Effect* = 0.4178, *SE* = 0.0211, *t* = 19.7898, *p* < .001, 95% CI = [0.3763, 0.4592]) and lower level of media locus of control (*Effect* = 0.2915, *SE* = 0.0268, *t* = 10.8976, *p* < .001, 95% CI = [0.2390, 0.3440]).

Finally, the direct effect of INE to radios on COVID-19 misperceptions was also significantly moderated by MLOC. Specifically, the 95% bias-corrected confidence intervals from 5,000 bootstrapped samples displayed a significant moderation model (*b* = 0.1538, *SE* = 0.0335, *t* = 4.5947, *p* < .001, 95% CI = [0.0881, 0.2196]). Figure 2.8 displays the interaction effect. Specifically, among those having greater perceived media locus of control, the effect of INE to radios on COVID-19 misperceptions became stronger (*Effect* = 0.3965, *SE* =

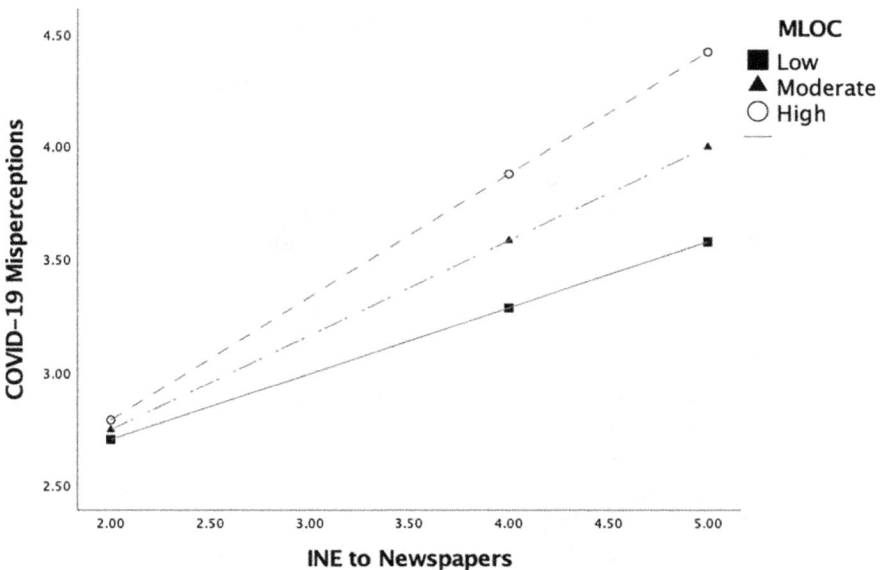

Figure 2.7 Two-way interaction between INE to newspapers and MLOC on COVID-19 misperceptions (US data).

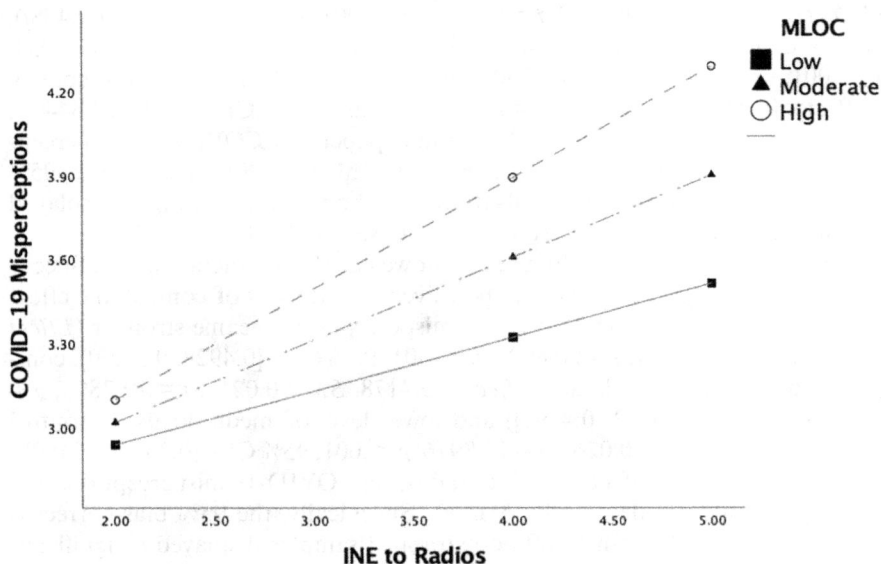

Figure 2.8 Two-way interaction between INE to radios and MLOC on COVID-19
        misperceptions (US data).

0.0266, *t* = 10.7981, *p* < .001, 95% CI = [0.2418, 0.3461]), compared to those
with moderate (*Effect* = 0.2939, *SE* = 0.0266, *t* = 11.0580, *p* < .001, 95% CI =
[0.2418, 0.3461]) and lower level of media locus of control (*Effect* = 0.1914, *SE*
= 0.0326, *t* = 5.8739, *p* < .001, 95% CI = [0.1274, 0.2553]). These findings al
imply that among those who believe that they have a good control of the news
they consume, the effects of INE on misperceptions were stronger.

When it comes to the moderating role of discussion network heterogeneity,
I applied the same analysis. Results of the 95% bias-corrected confidence intervals from 5,000 bootstrapped samples illustrated a significant moderation
model wherein discussion network heterogeneity moderated the main direct
effect of INE to TV on COVID-19 misperceptions (*b* = 0.1568, *SE* = 0.0262, *t*
= 5.9807, *p* < .001, 95% CI = [0.1053, 0.2083]). Figure 2.9 exhibits the interaction effect. Specifically, among those having higher level of discussion network
heterogeneity, the effect of INE to TV on COVID-19 misperceptions was
stronger (*Effect* = 0.5280, *SE* = 0.0328, *t* = 16.1108, *p* < .001, 95% CI = [0.4637,
0.5923]), compared to those with moderate (*Effect* = 0.4104, *SE* = 0.0256, *t* =
16.0046, *p* < .001, 95% CI = [0.3601, 0.4607]) and lower level of discussion
network heterogeneity (*Effect* = 0.3320, *SE* = 0.0284, *t* = 11.6689, *p* < .001,
95% CI = [0.2761, 0.3878]).

Additionally, same analysis was performed and the results of the 95%
bias-corrected confidence intervals from 5,000 bootstrapped samples again
showed a significant moderation model wherein discussion network heterogeneity moderated the main direct effect of INE to newspapers on COVID-19

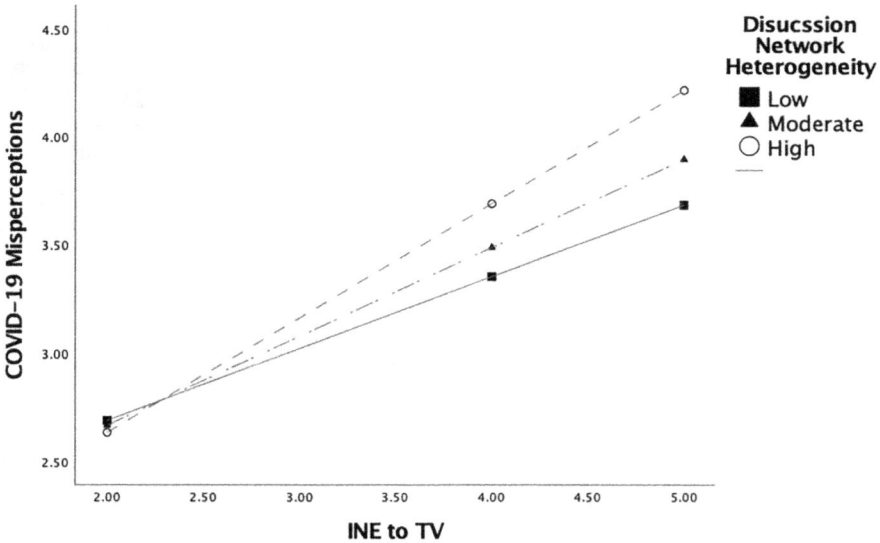

Figure 2.9 Two-way interaction between INE to TV and discussion network heterogeneity on COVID-19 misperceptions (US data).

misperceptions (b = 0.1550, SE = 0.0214, t = 7.2252, p < .001, 95% CI = [0.1129, 0.1970]). Figure 2.10 visualizes the interaction effect. Specifically, among those having higher level of discussion network heterogeneity, the effect of INE to newspapers on COVID-19 misperceptions was stronger (*Effect* = 0.5278, SE = 0.0254, t = 20.8101, p < .001, 95% CI = [0.4780, 0.5776]), compared to those with moderate (*Effect* = 0.4116, SE = 0.0217, t = 18.9796, p < .001, 95% CI = [0.3690, 0.4541]) and lower level of discussion network heterogeneity (*Effect* = 0.3341, SE = 0.0253, t = 13.1820, p < .001, 95% CI = [0.2844, 0.3838]).

Finally, Hayes' (2018) PROCESS macro model 1 was conducted to explore whether discussion network heterogeneity can also moderate the main direct effect of INE to radios on COVID-19 misperceptions. The results of the 95% bias-corrected confidence intervals from 5,000 bootstrapped samples showed that the interaction effect was not significant (b = 0.0257, SE = 0.0297, t = 0.8650, p = 0.3873, 95% CI = [−0.0326, 0.0841]). Figure 2.11 exhibits the insignificant interaction. These findings together showed that the extent of discussion network heterogeneity can only moderate the effects of INE to TV and newspapers on misperceptions, while it cannot moderate the effect of INE to radios.

Next, I analyze the Chinese data. As can be seen in Table 2.6, according to the hierarchical regression model, beyond all controls, among Chinese people, incidental news exposure to TV was not significantly associated with the factual knowledge of COVID-19 (b = 0.001, SE = 0.004, p = 0.904). Moreover,

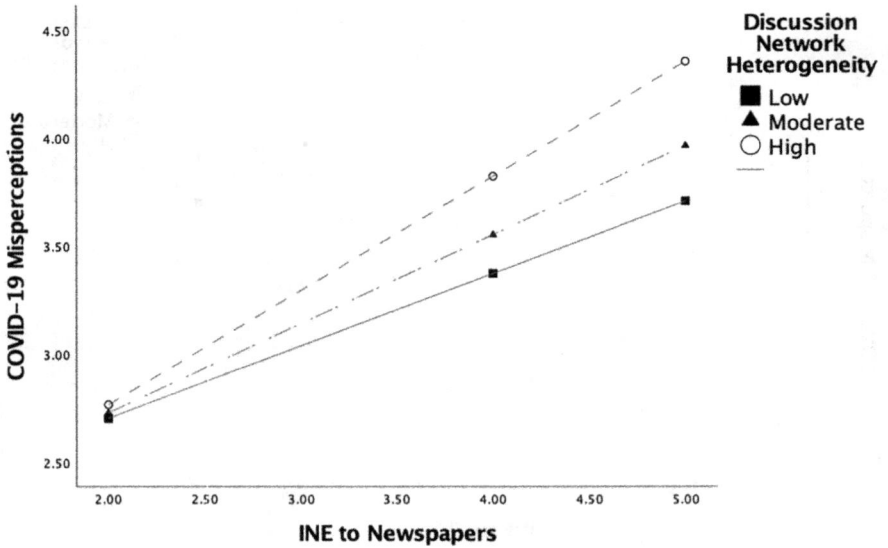

Figure 2.10 Two-way interaction between INE to newspapers and discussion network heterogeneity on COVID-19 misperceptions (US data).

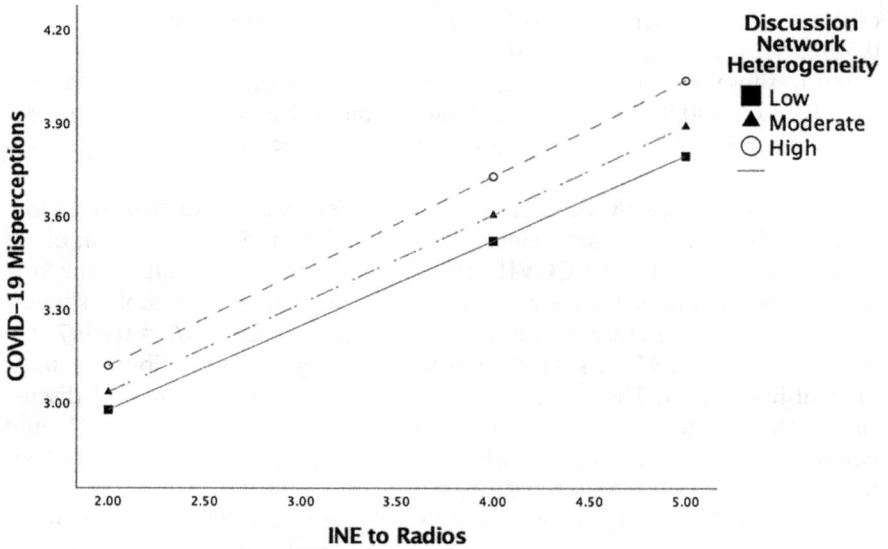

Figure 2.11 Two-way interaction between INE to radios and discussion network heterogeneity on COVID-19 misperceptions.

Table 2.6 Main direct effects of INE on COVID-19 knowledge level (Chinese data)

	COVID-19 Knowledge Level		
Step 1	*B*	*SE*	*t*
Constant	.63***	.05	13.14
Age	.000	.000	.26
Gender	−.002	.01	−.30
Education	.03***	.01	4.53
Monthly income	−.01†	.004	−1.93
News interest	.03***	.01	3.53
Political interest	.002	.01	.27
R^2	.18***		
Step 2			
Constant	.68***	.05	14.45
Age	.000	.000	.77
Gender	−.01	.01	−.61
Education	.02***	.01	4.13
Monthly income	−.01	.004	−1.37
News interest	.03***	.01	4.14
Political interest	.01	.01	1.07
INE to TV	.001	.004	.12
INE to newspapers	−.03***	.004	−6.17
INE to radio	−.01*	.004	−2.35
R^2	.29***		

Notes: Cell entries (b) are unstandardized betas. SE: Standard error. INE: incidental news exposure. † $p < .10$, *$p < .05$, **$p < .01$, ***$p < .001$.

incidental news exposure to newspapers also has significantly negative effects on the factual knowledge of COVID-19 ($b = -0.027$, $SE = 0.004$, $p < .001$). Similarly, incidental news exposure to radios also has a significantly negative impact on the factual knowledge of COVID-19 ($b = -0.009$, $SE = 0.004$, $p < 0.05$). These findings suggest that the more frequently individuals in China incidentally exposing themselves to news from newspapers and radios, the less likely they would develop better factual knowledge about the issue. This finding is in fact consistent with of what was shown in the U.S. sample.

Next, I add MLOC as a moderator in the three main associations. First, according to the output of PROCESS macro model 1, after controlling for all covariates, the result of the 95% bias-corrected confidence intervals from 5,000 bootstrapped samples demonstrated that among the Chinese individuals, the main association between INE to TV and the factual knowledge of COVID-19 was significantly moderated by individuals' media locus of control ($b = -0.0233$, *Boot SE* $= 0.0067$, $t = -3.4482$, $p < .001$, 95% CI $= [-0.0365, -0.0100]$). Figure 2.12 visualizes the interaction effect. Specifically, among those having greater perceived media locus of control, the effect of INE to TV on the factual knowledge of COVID-19 became lower (*Effect* $= -0.0270$, $SE = 0.0054$, $t = -5.0111$, $p < .001$, 95% CI $= [-0.03757, -0.0164]$), compared to those with moderate (*Effect* $= -0.0153$, $SE = 0.0041$, $t = -3.7015$, $p < .001$,

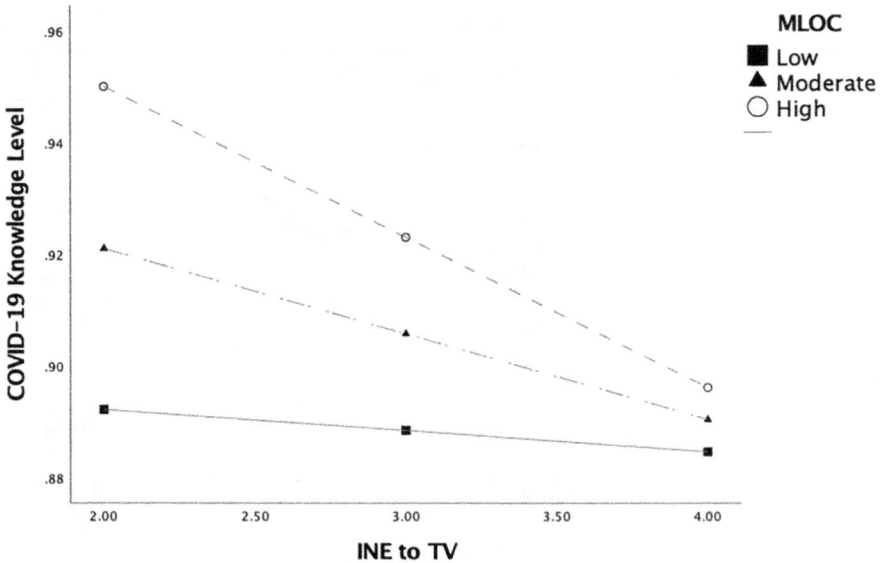

Figure 2.12 Two-way interaction between INE to TV and media locus of control on COVID-19 knowledge level (Chinese data).

95% CI = [−0.0235, −0.0072]) and lower level of media locus of control (*Effect* = −0.0037, *SE* = 0.0053, t = −0.7014, p = .48, 95% CI = [−0.0141, 0.0067]).

Further, the main association between INE to newspapers and the factual knowledge of COVID-19 was not significantly moderated by MLOC. Specifically, according to the output of PROCESS macro model 1, after controlling for all covariates, the result of the 95% bias-corrected confidence intervals from 5,000 bootstrapped samples demonstrated that among the Chinese individuals, MLOC did not interact with INE to newspapers to the factual knowledge of COVID-19 (b = 0.0069, *Boot SE* = 0.0161, t = 0.8935, p = 0.2710, 95% CI = [−0.0054, 0.0193]). Figure 2.13 visualizes the non-significant interaction.

Further, the main association between INE to radios and the factual knowledge of COVID-19 was also not significantly moderated by MLOC. Specifically, according to the output of PROCESS macro model 1, after controlling for all covariates, the result of the 95% bias-corrected confidence intervals from 5,000 bootstrapped samples demonstrated that among the Chinese individuals, MLOC did not interact with INE to radios to influence the factual knowledge of COVID-19 (b = 0.0030, *Boot SE* = 0.0061, t = 0.4952, p = 0.6206, 95% CI = [−0.0089, 0.0149]). Figure 2.14 visualizes the non-significant interaction.

Moreover, I investigate whether discussion network heterogeneity could also serve as a moderator to affect the main associations between INE to the three types of media on the factual knowledge of COVID-19. First, the main association between INE to TV and the factual knowledge of COVID-19 was

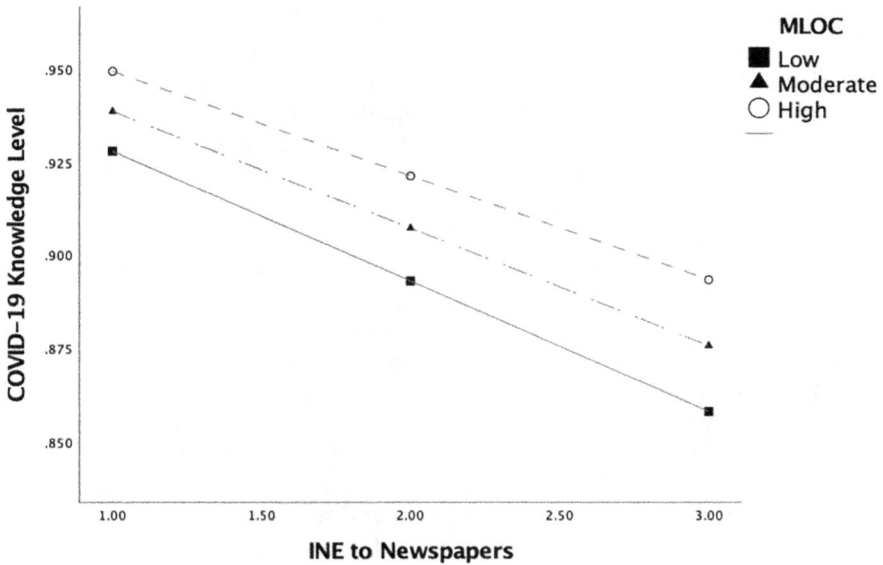

Figure 2.13 Two-way interaction between INE to newspapers and media locus of control on COVID-19 knowledge level (Chinese data).

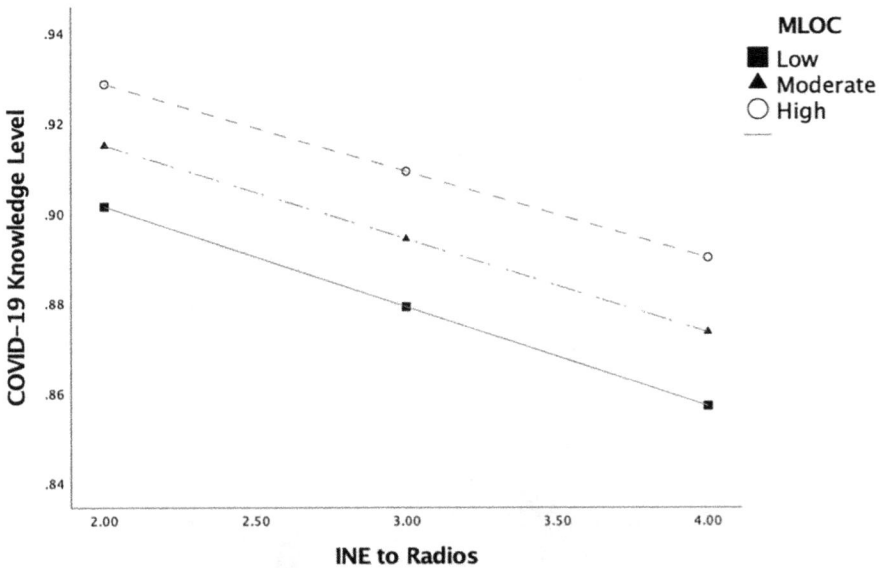

Figure 2.14 Two-way interaction between INE to radios and media locus of control on COVID-19 knowledge level (Chinese data).

not significantly moderated by discussion network heterogeneity. Specifically, according to the output of PROCESS macro model 1, after controlling for all covariates, the result of the 95% bias-corrected confidence intervals from 5,000 bootstrapped samples demonstrated that discussion network heterogeneity did not interact with INE to TV to influence the factual knowledge of COVID-19 ($b = -0.0051$, *Boot SE* $= 0.0052$, $t = -0.9961$, $p = 0.3194$, 95% CI $= [-0.0153, 0.0050]$). Figure 2.15 illustrates the non-significant interaction.

When it comes to the moderating effect of discussion network heterogeneity on the main association between INE to newspapers and the factual knowledge of COVID-19, according to the output of PROCESS macro model 1, after controlling for all covariates, the result of the 95% bias-corrected confidence intervals from 5,000 bootstrapped samples demonstrated that among the Chinese individuals, the main association between INE to newspapers and the factual knowledge of COVID-19 was significantly moderated by discussion network heterogeneity ($b = -0.0103$, *Boot SE* $= 0.0047$, $t = -2.2048$, $p < 0.05$, 95% CI $= [-0.0195, -0.0011]$). Figure 2.16 visualizes the significant interaction effect. Specifically, among those having greater discussion network heterogeneity, the effect of INE to newspapers on the factual knowledge of COVID-19 became lower (*Effect* $= -0.0298$, *SE* $= 0.0046$, $t = -6.4576$, $p < .001$, 95% CI $= [-0.0389, -0.0208]$), compared to those with moderate (*Effect* $= -0.0221$, *SE* $= 0.0040$, $t = -5.5324$, $p < .001$, 95% CI $= [-0.0300, -0.0143]$) and lower level of discussion network heterogeneity (*Effect* $= -0.0170$, *SE* $= 0.0051$, $t = -3.3260$, $p < .001$, 95% CI $= [-0.0270, -0.0070]$).

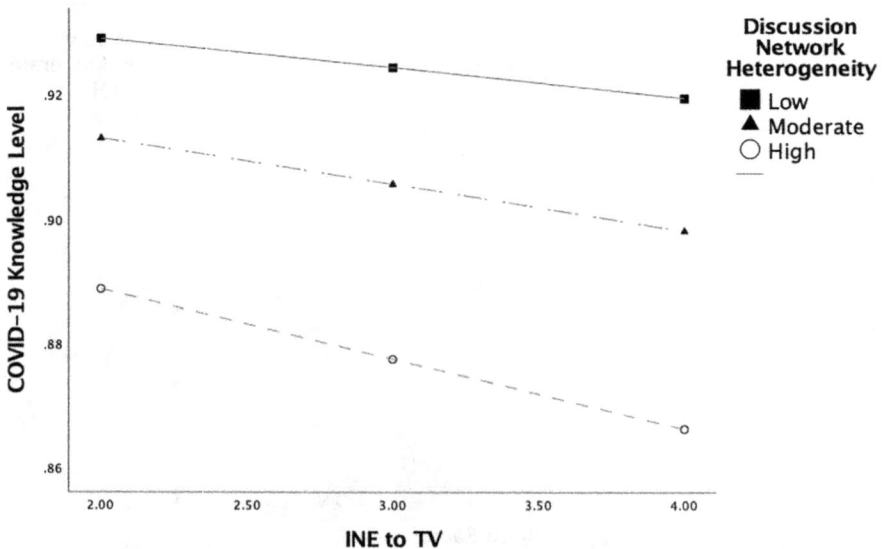

Figure 2.15 Two-way interaction between INE to TV and discussion network heterogeneity on COVID-19 knowledge level (Chinese data).

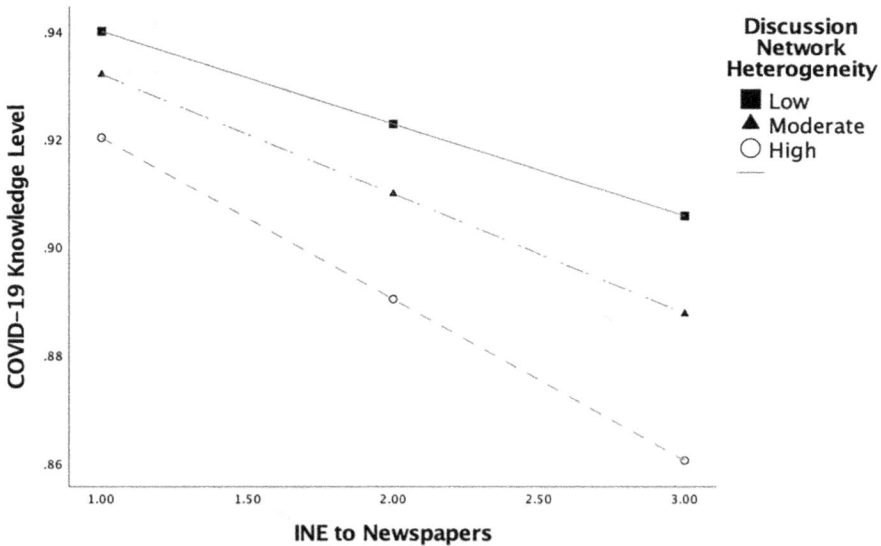

Figure 2.16 Two-way interaction between INE to newspapers and discussion network heterogeneity on COVID-19 knowledge level (Chinese data).

In terms of the moderating effect of discussion network heterogeneity on the main association between INE to radios and the factual knowledge of COVID-19, according to the output of PROCESS macro model 1, upon controlling for all covariates, the result of the 95% bias-corrected confidence intervals from 5,000 bootstrapped samples demonstrated that among the Chinese individuals, the main association between INE to radios and the factual knowledge of COVID-19 was significantly moderated by discussion network heterogeneity ($b = -0.0127$, *Boot SE* = 0.0048, $t = -2.6528$, $p < 0.01$, 95% CI = [-0.0222, -0.0033]). Figure 2.17 visualizes the significant interaction effect. Specifically, among those having greater discussion network heterogeneity, the effect of INE to newspapers on the factual knowledge of COVID-19 became lower (*Effect* = -0.0224, *SE* = 0.0048, $t = -4.6395$, $p < .001$, 95% CI = [-0.0318, -0.0129]), compared to those with moderate (*Effect* = -0.0128, *SE* = 0.0037, $t = -3.4327$, $p < .001$, 95% CI = [-0.0201, -0.0055]) and lower level of discussion network heterogeneity (*Effect* = -0.0065, *SE* = 0.0047, $t = -1.3710$, $p = 0.1706$, 95% CI = [-0.0157, 0.0028]).

2.6.8 Conclusion and Discussion

This section mainly addresses how incidental exposure to information influences people's misperceptions. Although INE is already a truism in the field of communication research, most of the prior studies have mainly focused on whether this passive information consumptive style could influence people's

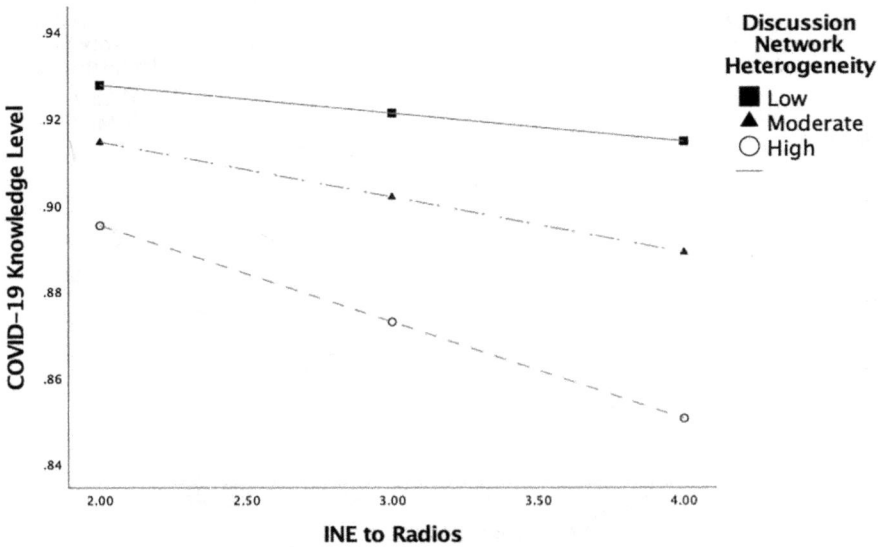

Figure 2.17 Two-way interaction between INE to radios and discussion network heterogeneity on COVID-19 knowledge level (Chinese data).

political participatory behavior and political knowledge level. Few studies have paid sufficient attention to the relationship between INE and people's misperceptions regarding major public health crises. However, I argue that this relationship is particularly worth discussing, because the COVID-19 pandemic has become an overriding issue for a few years. My argument is also underpinned by the concept of ambient news, which denotes the ubiquity and high rate of update of news and information (Hargreaves & Thomas, 2002). According to Gil de Zúñiga et al. (2022), the term "ambient" highlights that the perception is "developed peripherally" (p. 579). Undoubtedly, the COVID-19 pandemic has intensified such ambient news phenomenon, crystallizing and strengthening people's ambient awareness. Scholars highlighted that ambient news could create and facilitate individuals' false sense of media environment sophistication (Gil de Zúñiga et al., 2017). More worryingly, individuals' beliefs that they are well informed in this ambient news environment can represent a "psychological detachment" from active information seeking behavior (Gil de Zúñiga et al., 2017, p. 118). Therefore, the way people obtain information related to the pandemic has also gone beyond the single strategy of active searching or retrieval of information, instead, they rely more heavily on passive consumption or accidental exposure to the relevant information. Of course, in addition to the main effect of INE, individuals' media locus of control, discussion network heterogeneity, and defensive avoidance of information may also play a role in shaping the extent of misperceptions.

Findings in this section show that the more frequently individuals incidentally exposing themselves to traditional news media, the more likely they would have greater misperceptions regarding the pandemic or would exhibit lower level of factual knowledge about the pandemic. This finding provides new insights into the existing research on the effects of INE. Prior studies exhibited that INE can sometimes make people informed, while in my research, INE did not make people truly informed. Similar findings have emerged in Borah and associates' (2022) research, which demonstrated that INE to social media facilitated people's general misperceptions and COVID-19-related misperceptions, while little evidence has shown that INE to traditional media could also enhance misperceptions.

There are several possible explanations. First, the highly politicized nature of the COVID-19 pandemic makes it difficult for traditional media to guarantee the reliability and authentication of the relevant information they provide (Borah et al., 2023ab; Havey, 2020; Luengo & García-Marín, 2020; Su et al., 2022; Zhang et al., 2023). This point has already been discussed in one of the previous sections on the influence of partisan media use. In other words, although many people are optimistic about the role of traditional mass media in gatekeeping, suggesting that they are far less likely to become a misinformation hub, the fact is that traditional media have actually been lackluster during the time of COVID-19, and even contributed to partisan discourses and facilitated politicized agendas. The second potential reason may lie in the fact that due to the lack of surveillance motivation, those who often use a passive news consumption strategy may not generally prefer cognitively elaborating on the information they are exposed to because of the enormous cognitive costs involved, rendering no positive effect on learning and knowledge acquisition.

Besides, what is more interesting is that similar findings appeared in both contexts of the United States and China. This finding is of great significance for the enrichment and development of the theory because it shows that the negative effect of INE on knowledge acquisition and the positive effect of INE on misperceptions do not vary across both countries. These findings also reveal that the debate over the effects of INE is far from conclusive. Therefore, I call on future scholars to focus more on the effects of INE, especially its impact on people's cognition and knowledge levels. Given today's ambient news environment (Gil de Zúñiga et al., 2017; Hermida, 2010; Meraz & Papacharissi, 2013; Papacharissi, 2015), such passive information consumptive style is bound to become more common and ubiquitous.

In addition to the main effects of INE on misperceptions and factual knowledge, the conditional and indirect mechanisms are equally worthy of attention and discussion. In the analysis of the U.S. sample, the significant mediating effect of defensive avoidance buttressed my previous argument that INE may lead to avoidance rather than further involvement of news or cognitive elaboration of information. When it comes to MLOC, findings showed that in the U.S. context, MLOC was a positive moderator, namely, among those with greater MLOC, the positive effect of INE to the three types of traditional mass media on COVID-19 misperceptions became stronger. In other words, the more people perceive themselves as having a good control over their own information environment, the more likely they are to be influenced by INE to have stronger misperceptions. This finding is not incomprehensible. People with strong perceived MLOC may not elaborate more on the information that they incidentally exposed to, instead they may only pay sufficient attention and devote more cognitive efforts to the information obtained through their proactive curation. This may allow the misinformation to which they accidentally exposed take advantage of the situation, thereby eroding people's belief systems. Admittedly, this speculation still warrants further validation, future scholars could consider using qualitative methodologies such as focus groups or in-depth interviews to further understand other latent psychological factors. While in China, similarly significant moderation effect of MLOC was found in the main relationship between INE to TV and COVID-19 knowledge. The main effects of INE to newspapers and radio was not moderated by MLOC. These differential effects are understandable. In China, the functionality of hard news dissemination of radios and newspapers in China have become much less prominent, instead both outlets are committed to propagating policy information and providing entertainment.

Besides, findings also exhibited the significant moderating role of discussion network heterogeneity. However, contrary to previous studies, this study shows that among those of a higher level of discussion network heterogeneity, the positive effect of INE on misperceptions became stronger. A bulk of studies have shown that discussion network heterogeneity is a silver lining in the era of misinformation, significantly reducing people's misperceptions (Gill & Rojas, 2020; Su, 2021; Su et al., 2022), while this study has lent opposite evidence. This is likely because discussion network heterogeneity may not always serve as an endogenous variable in that it is in fact quite difficult for people to independently choose and curate their own social networks. Specifically, in many cases, people are forced to enter a certain social network, hence, their discussion network heterogeneity is not the result of their active choices and curations. In other words, even if a person is objectively in a highly heterogeneous social network, it does not always mean that he or she enjoys frequent exposure to diversified viewpoints or discussions with individuals of different socioeconomic status and social classes. Of course, this speculation can only explicate why discussion network heterogeneity does not play a positive role in reducing misperceptions, it can hardly explain the opposite moderation effect as shown in my findings. Therefore, qualitative investigations are quite imperative to unravel the potential mechanisms.

2.7 The News-Finds-Me Perception and Political Interest

2.7.1 The News-Finds-Me Perception

As reviewed above, the modern media environment in which different media compete for the public's attention has already rendered previous research in the direct effects of information consumption inadequate to capture the ever-changing media landscape and the shifting public psychology. In response to this high-choice news environment (Hameleers & Van der Meer, 2020; Hermida, 2010; Karlsen et al., 2020; Mangold & Bachl, 2018; Van Aelst et al., 2017), people tend to "take cues about what is, and what is not important from their extended social networks" (Gil de Zúñiga et al., 2019, p. 1257). The "news-finds-me" (NFM) perception is thus fostered. The incidental news exposure examined in the section above refers to the ways in which individuals exposed to information, while the NFM perception denotes modern news consumers' confidence in their own awareness of current affairs and the information accessibility in their networks, and relies on peripheral and heuristic, rather than central and active information processing (Gil de Zúñiga et al., 2017, 2019). In a nutshell, INE describes the behavior of news exposure without focusing on the perceptual dimension of individuals whereas the NFM perception indicates the confidence in getting informed without active surveillance of news (Gil de Zúñiga et al., 2017, 2019; Goyanes et al., 2023; Haim et al., 2021).

The NFM perception has become more prominent and ubiquitous because of today's networked, high-choice media environment in which people's attitudes have shifted from actively seeking for news from traditional media outlets toward waiting for their peers in social networks to inform them about current affairs (Gil de Zúñiga & Diehl, 2019). People have become more confident that they can be well informed even without actively monitoring the news. This kind of confidence is hinged not only upon the fact that media are competing for public's attentions, as I have mentioned above, but also upon the mechanism information is constantly updated on various media outlets and is notified to their audiences without a limitation of appointment (Gil de Zúñiga & Diehl, 2019; Hermida, 2010; Levordashka & Utz, 2016), not to mention that people's social networks are also growing stronger due to the generalization of weak ties (Gallos et al., 2012; Shen & Gong, 2019). In other words, people have been increasingly relying on the notification mechanisms of news media to inform them about current affairs and breaking news, while being less accustomed to satisfying their news needs only through actively searching for the news. When people find that they have never missed any important event just because they do not actively search for news, their NFM perception would become more solidified, and their reliance on the news media and social networks would also be intensified.

A broadly confirmed and adopted definition of the NFM perception is "[emphasis added] the extent to which individuals believe they can indirectly stay informed about public affairs – despite not actively following the news – through general Internet use, information received from peers, and connections within online social networks" (Gil de Zúñiga et al., 2017, p. 107). When it comes to the operationalization of the NFM perception, Song and associates (2020) suggested that the concept consists of three dimensions, namely, (1) the epistemic dimension, which denotes individuals' confidence that they can be well informed, (2) the motivational dimension, which indicates that individuals believe they do not need to seek for news, and (3) the instrumental dimension, which refers to individuals' reliance on peers in their social networks. Specifically, the epistemic dimension refers to the epistemic belief held by people that they have sufficient information. This dimension focuses on an outcome, namely, the state of knowing, rather than the means and channels through which this outcome is achieved. The motivational dimension, however, can be regarded as a further consequence of the epistemic dimension. That is, once individuals feel that they are already fully informed and are always in a state of knowing, they would not further actively follow the news with any explicit endeavors. The instrumental dimension describes the channel through which people achieve the above two dimensions. That is, through relying on peers, people get informed of current affairs and breaking news. This tripartite entails the internal factor structure of the NFM perception measurement, which has also been extensively utilized to operationalize the NFM perception as a variable in a bulk of subsequent research (Gil de Zúñiga & Diehl, 2019; Gil de Zúñiga et al., 2017, 2019; Goyanes et al., 2023).

In light of the literature reviewed above, it is safe to say that NFM demonstrates a disposition of passive news consumption, which is of low-effort cognitive style and involves people's peripheral or heuristic information processing, with low motivations to carefully scrutinize and elaborate on the information (Huang & Boukes, 2022; Lee et al., 2022; Razak & Sabarudin, 2023).

Plenty of empirical evidence regarding the effect of the NFM perception on individuals' perceptions, attitudes, and behaviors has been rendered. For instance, studies have demonstrated that the use of social media can facilitate the NFM perception (e.g., Gil de Zúñiga et al., 2022; Song et al., 2020). This is because in a highly saturated environment, obtaining information about current affairs does not require much active effort due to abundant information availability (Elenbaas et al., 2013; Prior, 2005). Against this backdrop, knowledge acquisition can occur without political motivation, interest in certain news, or necessary attention to certain contents (Bode, 2016; Shehata, 2014; Song et al., 2020). Gil de Zúñiga et al. (2022) also indicated that the NFM perception thrives by embedding in the current news ecosystem, revealing a positive path from social media news use to the NFM perception, which in turn triggered people's preference on algorithmic news. The rise and popularity of digital communication technologies has undermined and eroded the traditional role of gatekeepers that journalists have been playing (Nechushtai & Lewis, 2019), bringing forth a brand-new form of gatekeeping mechanism that is based upon artificial intelligence. A Newman report has documented that over half of new users worldwide reported preference of algorithm news over news edited, gatekept, or curated by journalism professionals (Newman et al., 2019). This undoubtedly proves that digital media has fully activated the initiative of people by providing rich technological affordances and realized its identity transfer from passive audience to active users able to generate content and curate consumptive feeds. In the current news-rich digital media environment, algorithmic news satisfies the information needs of individuals by prioritizing the most relevant information to them (Gil de Zúñiga et al., 2022).

Against this backdrop, most of the empirical studies have demonstrated a series of adverse democratic consequences of the NFM perception. For instance, Song and associates (2020) reported that people of greater NFM perception also exhibited higher preference to political cynicism. Strauß et al. (2021) suggested that individuals with an NFM perception exhibited a relatively low knowledge level and low critical cognitive resources necessary to evaluate news information. Similarly, Diehl and Lee (2021) found that individuals with a higher level of NFM perception were prone to incorrectly evaluate the credibility of fake news. Gil de Zúñiga et al. (2022) found that the NFM perception predicted political homophily. In other words, the over-reliance on one's social networks or media outlets could facilitate the development of homogeneous information and discussion political networks, which would undermine a deliberative democracy whose basic elements are the free flow of information and benign criticism. In general, we can infer through these empirical studies that people with higher NFM perception were less likely to utilize their cognitive resources to process and elaborate on information, therefore, they are more easily to be found in social media echo chambers than those with lower level of NFM perception. This also explains why high-NFM individuals exhibited lower expectancies of journalism quality (Segado-Boj et al., 2019, 2020), consumer fewer news from traditional media outlets (Park & Kaye, 2020), and demonstrated lower interest in politics and news (Gil de Zúñiga & Diehl, 2019).

In the current section I attempt to explore the relationship between the NFM perception and two outcomes, COVID-19 misperceptions and COVID-19 knowledge level, in the U.S. and China, respectively. I argue that it is imperative to study the NFM perception in the context of the pandemic, given one of the prerequisites for the construction of the NFM is the current high-choice news environment, and as I have mentioned earlier, information related to the pandemic is flooding various media and platforms, which not only gave birth to the ambient news but also contributed to the unique landscape of the "infodemic" (Eysenbach, 2020; Zarocostas, 2020). Therefore, I deem it necessary to revisit the effect of the NFM perception in the context of the COVID-19 pandemic. This attempt would ideally elucidate the mechanisms that influence misperceptions and knowledge levels in terms of information consumption patterns and perceptions of news.

2.7.2 Political Interest

Besides the main associations between the NFM perception and the COVID-19 misperceptions and knowledge level, I also attempt to investigate whether people's political interest could function as a moderator. One reason that I incorporate political interest into the regression model pertains to the argument in the prior literature that those high in the NFM perception are typically less interested in politics. Therefore, I attempt to investigate whether this is the case.

Scholars indicated that political sophistication is premised on one's political interest (Kruikemeier & Shehata, 2017; Lecheler & de Vreese, 2017). In other words, the extent to which an individual has knowledge of political activity and issues, assimilates information, and forms political viewpoints is stably hinged upon his or her interest in politics. In general, if a person has a strong and sustained interest in political issues, the person will typically satisfy their interest by actively following relevant news instead of waiting the news to find them. For example, when an individual does not have enough political interest, they may accept any information they come across accidentally and follow the guidance in the information; while if an individual has a strong interest in politics, even if they are passively exposed to massive amount of information, it is still possible that they go back to the source to validate its authenticity, elaborate on the information, and process the information cognitively and effortfully. Therefore, in the following data analysis, I would like to see whether the extent to which the NFM perception is associated with COVID-19 misperceptions and knowledge level is contingent upon people's political interests.

2.7.3 Methodology

The samples I used for analysis in this section are the same with those used in the prior sections. Specifically, upon removal of incomplete and invalid cases, the U.S. sample comprises 915 valid cases and the Chinese sample comprises 1333 valid cases. Detailed information regarding sampling procedures can be retrieved in the section above.

2.7.3.1 Measurements

NFM perception. In both the U.S. and the Chinese surveys, NFM perception was measured by asking the respondents to indicate the extent to which they agree with three statements, "I don't worry about keeping up with the news because I know news will find me," "I do not have to actively seek news because when important public affairs break, they will get to me through social media." and "I rely on information from my friends based on what they like or follow through social media" via a 5-point Likert scale (1 = never, 5 = always; $M_{U.S.} = 3.84$, $SD_{U.S.} = 0.81$, $\alpha_{U.S.} = 0.75$; $M_{China} = 3.27$, $SD_{China} = 0.70$, $\alpha_{U.S.} = 0.65$).

COVID-19 misperceptions (the U.S. sample). The measurement of the COVID-19 misperceptions consists of nine items. Each item was a piece of misinformation or conspiracy theory, and the respondents were asked to indicate the extent to which they agree with each statement on a 5-point Likert scale (1 = strongly disagree, 5 = strongly agree). The statements include "COVID-19 death rates are inflated," "Wearing a mask does not protect you from COVID-19," "5G radiant is the real cause of COVID-19," "Bill Gates intends to implant microchips in people via COVID-19 vaccination," and so forth. What needs to be reiterated is that misinformation and conspiracy theories do not necessarily mean that the message is fake, it highlights that the information per se lacks scientific evidence and can facilitate the devastation of the "infodemic" (Himelboim et al., 2023). The measurement of this variable reached satisfactory internal reliability ($M =$ 3.47, $SD = 1.09$, $\alpha = 0.95$).

COVID-19 knowledge level (the Chinese sample). Adapted from prior research (Austin et al., 2021), knowledge about COVID-19 was measured with true-or-false statements, with correct answers totalled, based on information from the World Health Organization (2020), the Centres for Disease Control and Prevention (2020), and a contemporary RTI (2020) survey. Respondents were asked to select true or false for the following seven statements: "Antibiotics can be used to treat the COVID-19 virus." "People of all ages can become infected with the COVID-19." "People of all ethnic groups can become infected with the COVID-19." "Eating garlic can lower your chances of getting infected with the COVID-19 virus." "Most people who are infected with COVID-19 virus die from it." "Most people who are infected with the COVID-19 virus recover from it." And "Older adults or those with compromised immune systems are at a higher risk" ($M = .90$, $SE = .16$, $\alpha = .88$).

Political interest. In both the U.S. and the Chinese surveys, political interest was assessed by the asking the respondents to indicate the extent to which they agree with one single item, "How interested, if at all, would you say you are in politics?" via a 5-point Likert scale ($M_{U.S.} = 3.71$, $SD_{U.S.} = 1.07$; $M_{China} = 3.83$, $SD_{China} = 0.64$).

Control variables. Akin to the above sections, I included control variables into the models to remove the concern of spurious effects. The controls included age ($M_{U.S.} = 37.47$, $SD_{U.S.} = 11.07$; $M_{China} = 37.64$, $SD_{China} = 11.29$), gender (U.S.: 44% female, 56% male; China: female: 55.4%, male: 44.6%), race (79.5% White, 20.5% non-whites), education ($Median_{U.S.} = 5$ [Bachelor's degree], $SD_{U.S.} = 0.83$), monthly income ($Median_{U.S.} = 4$ [\$8000-\$10,000], $SD = 1.61$; $Median_{China} = 3$ [10,0000–30,0000 CNY], $SD_{China} = 1.06$), Party ID (1 = strong Republican, 5 = strong Democrat; $M = 3.29$, $SD = 1.53$), and interest in news ($M_{U.S.} = 3.90$, $SD_{U.S.} = 1.06$; $M_{China} = 3.92$, $SD_{China} = 0.81$). Similar to the section above, race and Party ID were only used as control variables in the U.S. sample because both factors do not apply in China.

2.7.3.2 Analytical Strategy

In this section, I utilized Hayes' (2018) PROCESS macro model 1 to investigate the main association between NFM perception and COVID-19 misperceptions and knowledge level, as well as the moderation effect of political interest on the main relationships.

2.7.4 Results

I first analysed the U.S. data. According to the PROCESS macro model 1, findings in Table 2.7 exhibited that beyond all controls, there is a significant positive relationship between NFM perception and COVID-19 misperceptions among the U.S. respondents ($b = 0.86$, $SE = 0.13$, $t = 6.47$, $p < .001$, 95% CI: [0.5955, 1.1144]).

Table 2.7 Predictors of COVID-19 Misperceptions (U.S. data)

COVID-19 Misperceptions				
Step 1	B	SE	t	95% CI
Constant	1.93***	.58	3.36	[.8044, 3.0645]
Age	−.004	.003	−1.58	[−.0098, .0011]
Gender	−.35***	.06	−5.94	[−.4664, −.2346]
Race	−.24***	.02	−10.94	[−.2863, −.1992]
Education	−.28***	.04	−6.60	[−.3648, −.1976]
Monthly income	.22***	.02	10.71	[.1796, .2602]
Party ID	−.10***	.02	−4.90	[−.1386, −.0593]
News interest	.12**	.04	2.97	[.0393, .1924]
Step 2				
NFM perception	.86***	.13	6.47	[.5955, 1.1144]
NFM perception × Political interest	−.13***	.03	−4.78	[−.1932, 0.0611]
R^2	.38***			

Notes: Cell entries (b) are unstandardized betas. SE: Standard error. INE: incidental news exposure. 95% CI: with lower-level confidence interval and upper-level confidence interval in brackets. *$p < .05$, **$p < .01$, ***$p < .001$.

When it comes to the moderation effect, results of the PROCESS macro model 1 suggests that there is a significant negative two-way interaction between NFM perception and political interest on COVID-19 misperceptions ($b = -0.13$, $SE = 0.03$, $t = -3.78$, $p < .001$, 95% CI: [−0.1932, −0.0611]). Approximately 38% of the variance in COVID-19 misperceptions was accounted for by the predictors ($R^2 = .38$). As can be seen in Figure 2.18, among those with a higher level of political interest, the main association between NFM perception and COVID-19 misperceptions became weaker (*Effect* = 0.2193, $SE = 0.0583$, $t = 3.7643$, $p < .001$, 95% CI = [0.1050, 0.3336]), compared to those of a moderate (*Effect* = 0.3464, $SE = 0.0410$, $t = 8.4520$, $p < .001$, 95% CI = [0.2660, 0.4269]) and a lower level of political interest (*Effect* = 0.4736, $SE = 0.0472$, $t = 10.0264$, $p < .001$, 95% CI = [0.3809, 0.5663]).

Next, I analyzed the Chinese data. According to the PROCESS macro model 1, findings in Table 2.8 exhibited that beyond all controls, there is a significant negative relationship between NFM perception and COVID-19 knowledge level among the Chinese respondents ($b = -0.07$, $SE = 0.30$, $t = -2.21$, $p < .05$, 95% CI: [−0.1243, −0.0073]). When it comes to the moderating role of political interest, model 1 shows that the interaction is not significant ($b = 0.01$, $SE = 0.01$, $t = 1.64$, $p = 0.10$, 95% CI: [−0.0023, 0.0261]).

2.7.5 Conclusion and Discussion

With the popularity of digital communication technologies and the emergence of the ambient news environment, people have shifted from actively seeking for what they are interested in through news media, toward passively waiting for

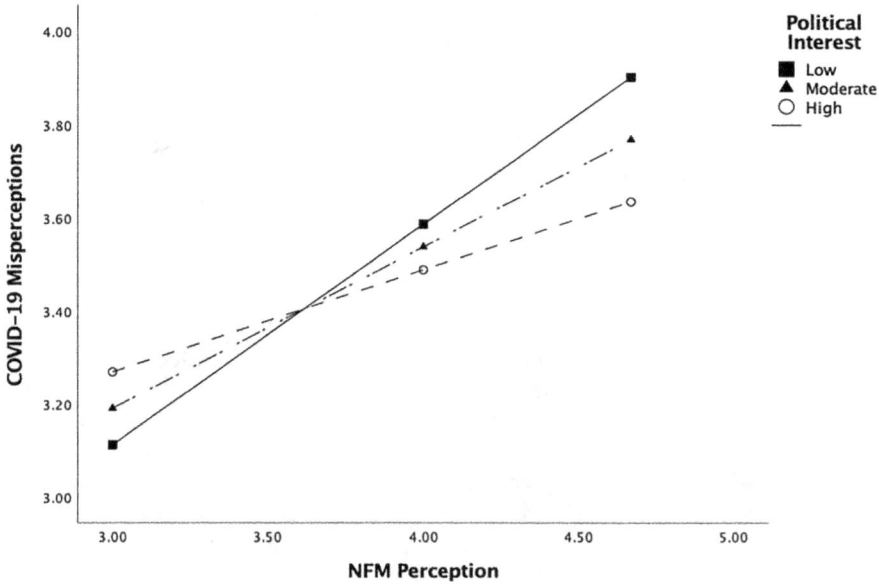

Figure 2.18 Two-way interaction between NFM perception and political interest on COVID-19 misperceptions (U.S. data).

Table 2.8 Predictors of Factual Knowledge of COVID-19 (Chinese data)

	COVID-19 Knowledge Level			
Step 1	*B*	*SE*	*t*	*95% CI*
Constant	.83***	.10	8.18	[.6356, 1.0364]
Age	−.0004	.001	−.80	[−.0015, .0006]
Gender	−.002	.01	−.23	[−.0184, .0144]
Education	.03***	.01	4.45	[.0153, .0394]
Monthly income	−.01	.004	−1.78	[−.0161, .0008]
News interest	.03***	.01	3.69	[.0127, .0413]
Step 2				
NFM perception	−.07*	.03	−2.21	[−.1243, −.0073]
NFM perception × Political interest	.01	.01	1.64	[−.0023, .0261]
R^2	.04***			

Notes: Cell entries (b) are unstandardized betas. SE: Standard error. INE: incidental news exposure. 95% CI: with lower-level confidence interval and upper-level confidence interval in brackets. *$p < .05$, **$p < .01$, ***$p < .001$.

the news to find them. Prior studies have probed the consequences and ramifications of such NFM perception mainly in the realm of political communication, rendering rich evidence regarding how the NFM perception would undermine democracy, while what remains unknown pertains to whether such perception could also influence public understanding and knowledge of public health and scientific issues. Therefore, in this section, I examined the both the main associations between the NFM perception and the COVID-19 misperceptions and knowledge level and the role of political interest in moderating these main associations.

Findings demonstrated that the NFM perception was positively associated with COVID-19 misperceptions and was negatively associated with COVID-19 knowledge level. This finding implies that such passivity is indeed detrimental to the understanding of public affairs and may even provide a good basis for the spread of misinformation. The traditional Cognitive Mediation Model (CMM) suggests that surveillance of news can induce active news seeking and attention, which further triggers cognitive elaboration, in turn facilitating learning (Evelande Jr., 2001). Hence, it is easily inferred that people's motivation, surveillance need, and active seeking behavior are irreplaceably important predispositions of knowledge acquisition (Beaudoin & Thorson, 2004; Jensen, 2011). This explains the underlying factors that contribute to the negative effect of NFM perception on COVID-19 knowledge and the positive effect of it on COVID-19 misperceptions.

In fact, this finding has strong practical significance. Integrating the findings of this section and the results of some previous empirical studies (e.g., Gil de Zúñiga et al., 2022), we should be fully cognizant of the adverse consequences of the NFM perception a democratic society and an informed public. We can imagine a scenario under which every individual has a fairly high level of NFM perception, if so, nobody would actively seek for information in a proactive way. Hence, people's perception of reality and formation of knowledge structures would be entirely determined by the algorithm and their social networks. In other words, once individuals give up their rights to actively seek for information and curate their consumptive news feeds, the algorithm mechanism of social media platforms will inevitably be empowered to shape and dominate human perceptions. Although this scenario is somewhat absolute, we have to be vigilant against it.

According to my analysis results, political interest has played a significant moderating role in the context of the U.S., while it was not a significant moderator in the Chinese context. Specifically, in the U.S., among those with a stronger interest in politics, the positive tie between the NFM perception and COVID-19 misperceptions became weaker. This finding suggests that political interest might be a silver lining preventing those passive populations from falling for misinformation. This also echoes previous findings regarding the positive relationship between interest and consumptive news feeds curation (Lee et al., 2019; Lu, 2020; Merten, 2021). In terms of the null effect of political interest in the context of China, this might be attributed to the fact that in a tight media environment, people's political interest does not always lead to access to and retrieval of more and complex information, nor does it necessarily contribute to a higher extent of political sophistication.

References

Ahmed, S., & Gil-Lopez, T. (2022). Incidental news exposure on social media and political participation gaps: Unraveling the role of education and social networks. *Telematics and Informatics*, *68*, 101764.

Ahmed, W., Vidal-Alaball, J., Downing, J., & Seguí, F. L. (2020). COVID-19 and the 5G conspiracy theory: Social network analysis of Twitter data. *Journal of Medical Internet Research*, *22*(5), e19458.

Allcott, H., Boxell, L., Conway, J., Gentzkow, M., Thaler, M., & Yang, D. (2020). Polarization and public health: Partisan differences in social distancing during the coronavirus pandemic. *Journal of Public Economics*, *191*, 104254.

Amazeen, M. A. (2020). News in an era of content confusion: Effects of news use motivations and context on native advertising and digital news perceptions. *Journalism & Mass Communication Quarterly*, *97*(1), 161–187.

Amodio, D. M., Jost, J. T., Master, S. L., & Yee, C. M. (2007). Neurocognitive correlates of liberalism and conservatism. *Nature Neuroscience*, *10*(10), 1246–1247.

Anderson, J. T. L., Howell, E. L., Xenos, M. A., Scheufele, D. A., & Brossard, D. (2021). Learning without seeking? Incidental exposure to science news on social media & knowledge of gene editing. *Journal of Science Communication*, *20*(4), A01.

Austin, E. W., Austin, B. W., Willoughby, J. F., Amram, O., & Domgaard, S. (2021). How media literacy and science media literacy predicted the adoption of protective behaviors amidst the COVID-19 pandemic. *Journal of Health Communication*, *26*(4), 239–252.

Ardèvol-Abreu, A., Hooker, C. M., & Gil de Zúñiga, H. (2018). Online news creation, trust in the media, and political participation: Direct and moderating effects over time. *Journalism*, *19*(5), 611–631.

Austin, E. W., Muldrow, A. F., & Austin, B. W. (2016). Examining how media literacy and personality factors predict skepticism toward alcohol advertising. *Journal of Health Communication*, *21*(5), 600–609.

Ballew, M. T., Rosenthal, S. A., Goldberg, M. H., Gustafson, A., Kotcher, J. E., Maibach, E. W., & Leiserowitz, A. (2020). Beliefs about others' global warming beliefs: The role of party affiliation and opinion deviance. *Journal of Environmental Psychology*, *70*, 101466.

Baum, M. A. (2002). Sex, lies, and war: How soft news brings foreign policy to the inattentive public. *American Political Science Review*, *96*(1), 91–109.

Bayes, R., & Druckman, J. N. (2021). Motivated reasoning and climate change. *Current Opinion in Behavioral Sciences*, *42*, 27–35.

Beaudoin, C. E., & Thorson, E. (2004). Testing the cognitive mediation model: The roles of news reliance and three gratifications sought. *Communication Research*, *31*(4), 446–471.

Benegal, S. D., & Scruggs, L. A. (2018). Correcting misinformation about climate change: The impact of partisanship in an experimental setting. *Climatic Change*, *148*(1–2), 61–80.

Bennett, W. L., & Livingston, S. G. (2018). The disinformation order: Disruptive communication and the decline of democratic institutions. *European Journal of Communication*, *33*, 122–139.

Berinsky, A. J., Huber, G. A., & Lenz, G. S. (2012). Evaluating online labor markets for experimental research: Amazon.com's Mechanical Turk. *Political Analysis, 20*, 351–368.

Biasio, L. R. (2017). Vaccine hesitancy and health literacy. *Human Vaccines & Immunotherapeutics, 13*(3), 701–702.

Bicchieri, C., Fatas, E., Aldama, A., Casas, A., Deshpande, I., Lauro, M., ... Wen, R. (2021). In science we (should) trust: Expectations and compliance across nine countries during the COVID-19 pandemic. *PloS one, 16*(6), e0252892.

Boas, T. C., Christenson, D. P., & Glick, D. M. (2020). Recruiting large online samples in the United States and India: Facebook, mechanical turk, and qualtrics. *Political Science Research & Methods, 8*(2), 232–250.

Boczkowski, P. J., Mitchelstein, E., & Matassi, M. (2018). "News comes across when I'm in a moment of leisure": Understanding the practices of incidental news consumption on social media. *New Media & Society, 20*(10), 3523–3539.

Bode, L. (2016). Political news in the news feed: Learning politics from social media. *Mass Communication & Society, 19*(1), 24–48.

Bode, L., & Vraga, E. K. (2018). See something, say something: Correction of global health misinformation on social media. *Health Communication, 33*(9), 1131–1140.

Bolsen, T., Druckman, J. N., & Cook, F. L. (2014). The influence of partisan motivated reasoning on public opinion. *Political Behavior, 36*(2), 235–262.

Borah, P. (2022). The moderating role of political ideology: Need for cognition, media locus of control, misinformation efficacy, and misperceptions about COVID-19. *International Journal of Communication, 16*, 3534–3559.

Borah, P., Austin, E., & Su, Y. (2023b). Injecting disinfectants to kill the virus: Media literacy, information gathering sources, and the moderating role of political ideology on misperceptions about COVID-19. *Mass Communication & Society, 26*(4), 1–27.

Borah, P., Ghosh, S., Hwang, J., Shah, D. V., & Brauer, M. (2023a). Red media vs. blue media: Social distancing and partisan news media use during the COVID-19 pandemic. *Health Communication*, 1–11.

Borah, P., Su, Y., Xiao, X., & Lee, D. K. L. (2022). Incidental news exposure and COVID-19 misperceptions: A moderated-mediation model. *Computers in Human Behavior, 129*, 107173.

Bridgman, A., Merkley, E., Loewen, P. J., Owen, T., Ruths, D., Teichmann, L., & Zhilin, O. (2020). The causes and consequences of COVID-19 misperceptions: Understanding the role of news and social media. *Harvard Kennedy School Misinformation Review, 1*(3), 1–18.

Cacioppo, J. T., & Petty, R. E. (1982). The need for cognition. *Journal of Personality and Social Psychology, 42*(1), 116–131.

Cadeddu, C., Daugbjerg, S., Ricciardi, W., & Rosano, A. (2020). Beliefs towards vaccination and trust in the scientific community in Italy. *Vaccine, 38*(42), 6609–6617.

Calvillo, D. P., Ross, B. J., Garcia, R. J., Smelter, T. J., & Rutchick, A. M. (2020). Political ideology predicts perceptions of the threat of COVID-19 (and susceptibility to fake news about it). *Social Psychological and Personality Science, 11*(8), 1119–1128.

Carey, J. M., Guess, A. M., Loewen, P. J., Merkley, E., Nyhan, B., Phillips, J. B., & Reifler, J. (2022). The ephemeral effects of fact-checks on COVID-19 misperceptions in the United States, Great Britain and Canada. *Nature Human Behaviour, 6*(2), 236–243.

Centers for Disease Control and Prevention (2020). Symptoms of Coronavirus. Retrieved from March 13, 2020 https://www.cdc.gov/coronavirus/2019-ncov/symptoms-testing/symptoms.html

Chen, H.-T. (2021). Second screening and the engaged public: The role of second screening for news and political expression in an O-S-R-O-R model. *Journalism & Mass Communication Quarterly, 98*(2), 526–546.

Chen, H. T., Kim, Y., & Chan, M. (2022). Just a glance, or more? Pathways from counter-attitudinal incidental exposure to attitude (de) polarization through response behaviors and cognitive elaboration. *Journal of Communication, 72*(1), 83–110.

Chen, L., & Yang, X. (2019). Using EPPM to evaluate the effectiveness of fear appeal messages across different media outlets to increase the intention of breast self-examination among Chinese women. *Health Communication, 34*(11), 1369–1376.

Chen, L., Tang, H., Liao, S., & Hu, Y. (2021). E-health campaigns for promoting influenza vaccination: Examining effectiveness of fear appeal messages from different sources. *Telemedicine and e-Health, 27*(7), 763–770.

Chen, M., & Chen, L. (2021). Promoting smoking cessation in China: Using an expansion of the EPPM with other-oriented threat. *Journal of Health Communication, 26*(3), 174–183.

Chinn, S., & Pasek, J. (2021). Some deficits and some misperceptions: Linking partisanship with climate change cognitions. *International Journal of Public Opinion Research, 33*(2), 235–254.

Chinn, S., Hart, P. S., & Soroka, S. (2020). Politicization and polarization in climate change news content, 1985–2017. *Science Communication, 42*, 112–129.

Cho, H., & Salmon, C. T. (2006). Fear appeals for individuals in different stages of change: Intended and unintended effects and implications on public health campaigns. *Health Communication, 20*(1), 91–99.

Cho, J., Shah, D. V., McLeod, J. M., McLeod, D. M., Scholl, R. M., & Gotlieb, M. R. (2009). Campaigns, reflection, and deliberation: Advancing an O-S-R-O-R model of communication effects. *Communication Theory, 19*(1), 66–88.

Choi, H. (2022). How partisan cable news mobilizes viewers: Partisan media, discussion networks and political participation. *Journal of Broadcasting & Electronic Media, 66*(1), 129–152.

Chou, W. Y. S., & Budenz, A. (2020). Considering emotion in COVID-19 vaccine communication: Addressing vaccine hesitancy and fostering vaccine confidence. *Health Communication, 35*(14), 1718–1722.

Chung, M., & Jones-Jang, S. M. (2022). Red media, blue media, Trump briefings, and COVID-19: Examining how information sources predict risk preventive behaviors via threat and efficacy. *Health Communication, 37*(14), 1707–1714.

Cinelli, M., De Francisci Morales, G., Galeazzi, A., Quattrociocchi, W., & Starnini, M. (2021). The echo chamber effect on social media. *Proceedings of the National Academy of Sciences, 118*(9), e2023301118.

Conway III, L. G., Woodard, S. R., Zubrod, A., & Chan, L. (2021). Why are conservatives less concerned about the coronavirus (COVID-19) than liberals? Comparing political, experiential, and partisan messaging explanations. *Personality and Individual Differences, 183*, 111124.

Cuan-Baltazar, J. Y., Muñoz-Perez, M. J., Robledo-Vega, C., Pérez-Zepeda, M. F., & Soto-Vega, E. (2020). Misinformation of COVID-19 on the internet: Infodemiology study. *JMIR Public Health & Surveillance, 6*(2), e18444.

Dahlgren, P. (2005). The Internet, public spheres, and political communication: Dispersion and deliberation. *Political Communication, 22*(2), 147–162.

Dalege, J., & van der Does, T. (2022). Using a cognitive network model of moral and social beliefs to explain belief change. *Science Advances, 8*(33), eabm0137.

Denzau, A. D., & North, D. C. (1994). Shared mental models: Ideologies and institutions. In A. Lupia, M. C. McCubbins, & S. L. Popkin (Eds.), *Elements of reason: Cognition, choice, and the bounds of rationality* (pp. 23–46). New York: Cambridge University Press

Detoc, M., Bruel, S., Frappe, P., Tardy, B., Botelho-Nevers, E., & Gagneux-Brunon, A. (2020). Intention to participate in a COVID-19 vaccine clinical trial and to get vaccinated against COVID-19 in France during the pandemic. *Vaccine, 38*(45), 7002–7006.

Diehl, T., & Lee, S. (2021). News find Me perception and fake news credibility: Testing the cognitive involvement hypothesis on social media. *Computers in Human Behavior, 128*, 107121.

Downs, A. (1957). An economic theory of political action in a democracy. *Journal of Political Economy, 65*(2), 135–150.

Druckman, J. N., & McGrath, M. C. (2019). The evidence for motivated reasoning in climate change preference formation. *Nature Climate Change, 9*(2), 111–119.

Druckman, J. N., Ognyanova, K., Baum, M. A., Lazer, D., Perlis, R. H., Volpe, J. D., ... Simonson, M. (2021). The role of race, religion, and partisanship in misperceptions about COVID-19. *Group Processes & Intergroup Relations, 24*(4), 638–657.

Druckman, J. N., Peterson, E., & Slothuus, R. (2013). How elite partisan polarization affects public opinion formation. *American Political Science Review, 107*(1), 57–79.

Eisenstadt, S. N., Aizenshtadt, S. N., & Roniger, L. (1984). *Patrons, clients and friends: Interpersonal relations and the structure of trust in society.* Cambridge University Press.

Elenbaas, M., Boomgaarden, H. G., Schuck, A. R., & de Vreese, C. H. (2013). The impact of media coverage and motivation on performance-relevant information. *Political Communication, 30*(1), 1–16.

Enders, A. M., Uscinski, J. E., Klofstad, C., & Stoler, J. (2020). The different forms of COVID-19 misinformation and their consequences. *Harvard Kennedy School Misinformation Review*, 1–21.

Epstein, S., Pacini, R., Denes-Raj, V., & Heier, H. (1996). Individual differences in intuitive-experiential and analytical-rational thinking styles. *Journal of Personality and Social Psychology, 71*(2), 390–405.

Erikson, R. S., & Tedin, K. L., (2003). *American public opinion* (6th ed). New York: Longman.

Eveland Jr, W. P. (2001). The cognitive mediation model of learning from the news: Evidence from nonelection, off-year election, and presidential election contexts. *Communication Research, 28*(5), 571–601.

Eveland Jr., W. P., Shah, D. V., & Kwak, N. (2003). Assessing causality in the cognitive mediation model: A panel study of motivations, information processing, and learning during campaign 2000. *Communication Research, 30*(4), 359–386.

Eysenbach, G. (2020). How to fight an infodemic: The four pillars of infodemic management. *Journal of Medical Internet Research, 22*(6), e21820.

Farrell, J., McConnell, K., & Brulle, R. (2019). Evidence-based strategies to combat scientific misinformation. *Nature Climate Change, 9*(3), 191–195.

Federico, C. M., & Goren, P. (2009). Motivated social cognition and ideology: Is attention to elite discourse a prerequisite for epistemically motivated political affinities? In J. T. Jost, A. C. Kay, & H. Thorisdottir (Eds.), *Social and psychological bases of ideology and system justification* (pp. 267–291). Oxford University Press.

Feezell, J. T. (2018). Agenda setting through social media: The importance of incidental news exposure and social filtering in the digital era. *Political Research Quarterly, 71*(2), 482–494.

Feldman, L., Hart, P. S., & Milosevic, T. (2017). Polarizing news? Representations of threat and efficacy in leading US newspapers' coverage of climate change. *Public Understanding of Science, 26*(4), 481–497.

Feldman, L., Maibach, E. W., Roser-Renouf, C., & Leiserowitz, A. (2012). Climate on cable: The nature and impact of global warming coverage on Fox News, CNN, and MSNBC. *The International Journal of Press/Politics, 17*(1), 3–31.

Fletcher, R., & Nielsen, R. K. (2018). Are people incidentally exposed to news on social media? A comparative analysis. *New Media & Society, 20*(7), 2450–2468.

Flores, A., Cole, J. C., Dickert, S., Eom, K., Jiga-Boy, G. M., Kogut, T., … Van Boven, L. (2022). Politicians polarize and experts depolarize public support for COVID-19 management policies across countries. *Proceedings of the National Academy of Sciences, 119*(3), e2117543119.

Freiling, I., Krause, N. M., Scheufele, D. A., & Brossard, D. (2023). Believing and sharing misinformation, fact-checks, and accurate information on social media: The role of anxiety during COVID-19. *New Media & Society, 25*(1), 141–162.

Fukuyama, F (1995) *Trust: The Social Virtues and the Creation of Prosperity.* NY: Free Press.

Gadarian, S. K., Goodman, S. W., & Pepinsky, T. B. (2021). Partisanship, health behavior, and policy attitudes in the early stages of the COVID-19 pandemic. *Plos one, 16*(4), e0249596.

Gallos, L. K., Makse, H. A., & Sigman, M. (2012). A small world of weak ties provides optimal global integration of self-similar modules in functional brain networks. *Proceedings of the National Academy of Sciences, 109*(8), 2825–2830.

Garrett, R. K., Long, J. A., & Jeong, M. S. (2019). From partisan media to misperception: Affective polarization as mediator. *Journal of Communication, 69*(5), 490–512

Garrett, R. K., Weeks, B. E., & Neo, R. L. (2016). Driving a wedge between evidence and beliefs: How online ideological news exposure promotes political misperceptions. *Journal of Computer-Mediated Communication, 21*(5), 331–348.

Geiger, N., Gore, A., Squire, C. V., & Attari, S. Z. (2021). Investigating similarities and differences in individual reactions to the COVID-19 pandemic and the climate crisis. *Climatic Change, 167*(1–2), 1.

Goodwin, J., & Jasper, J. M. (2006). Emotions and social movements. In J. E. Stets & J. H. Turner (Eds.), *Handbook of the Sociology of Emotions.* Handbooks of Sociology and Social Research (pp. 611–636). Boston, MA: Springer.

Chaiken, S., Giner-Sorolla, R., & Chen, S. (1996). Beyond accuracy: Defense and impression motives in heuristic and systematic information processing. In P. M. Gollwitzer & J. A. Bargh (Eds.), *The psychology of action: Linking cognition and motivation to behavior* (pp. 553–578). The Guilford Press.

Galston, W. A. (2021, March 22). A momentous shift in US public attitudes toward China. *Brookings.* Retrieved from https://www.brookings.edu/blog/order-from-chaos/2021/03/22/a-momentous-shift-in-us-public-attitudes-toward-china/

Gil de Zúñiga, H., Borah, P., & Goyanes, M. (2021). How do people learn about politics when inadvertently exposed to news? Incidental news paradoxical Direct and indirect effects on political knowledge. *Computers in Human Behavior, 121*, 106803.

Gil de Zúñiga, H., Cheng, Z., & González-González, P. (2022). Effects of the News Finds Me perception on algorithmic news attitudes and social media political homophily. *Journal of Communication, 72*(5), 578–591.

Gil de Zúñiga, H., Correa, T., & Valenzuela, S. (2012). Selective exposure to cable news and immigration in the US: The relationship between FOX News, CNN, and attitudes toward Mexican immigrants. *Journal of Broadcasting & Electronic Media, 56*(4), 597–615.

Gil de Zúñiga, H., & Diehl, T. (2019). News finds me perception and democracy: Effects on political knowledge, political interest, and voting. *New Media & Society, 21*(6), 1253–1271.

Gil de Zúñiga, H., Diehl, T., Huber, B., & Liu, J. H. (2019). The citizen communication mediation model across countries: A multilevel mediation model of news use and discussion on political participation. *Journal of Communication, 69*(2), 144–167.

Gil de Zúñiga, H., Valenzuela, S., & Weeks, B. E. (2016). Motivations for political discussion: Antecedents and consequences on civic engagement. *Human Communication Research, 42*(4), 533–552.

Gil de Zúñiga, H., Weeks, B., & Ardèvol-Abreu, A. (2017). Effects of the news-finds-me perception in communication: Social media use implications for news seeking and learning about politics. *Journal of Computer-Mediated Communication, 22*(3), 105–123.

Gill, H., & Rojas, H. (2020). Chatting in a mobile chamber: Effects of instant messenger use on tolerance toward political misinformation among South Koreans. *Asian Journal of Communication, 30*(6), 470–493.

Gilad, B., Kaish, S., & Loeb, P. D. (1987). Cognitive dissonance and utility maximization: A general framework. *Journal of Economic Behavior & Organization, 8*(1), 61–73.

Goldenberg, M. J. (2016). Public misunderstanding of science? Reframing the problem of vaccine hesitancy. *Perspectives on Science, 24*(5), 552–581.

Goodall, C. E., & Reed, P. (2013). Threat and efficacy uncertainty in news coverage about bed bugs as unique predictors of information seeking and avoidance: An extension of the EPPM. *Health Communication, 28*(1), 63–71.

Gore, T. D., & Bracken, C. C. (2005). Testing the theoretical design of a health risk message: Reexamining the major tenets of the extended parallel process model. *Health Education & Behavior, 32*(1), 27–41.

Goyanes, M. (2020). Antecedents of incidental news exposure: The role of media preference, use and trust. *Journalism Practice, 14*(6), 714–729.

Goyanes, M., Ardèvol-Abreu, A., & Gil de Zúñiga, H. (2023). Antecedents of news avoidance: Competing effects of political interest, news overload, trust in news media, and "news finds me" perception. *Digital Journalism, 11*(1), 1–18.

Goyanes, M., & Demeter, M. (2022). Beyond positive or negative: Understanding the phenomenology, typologies and impact of incidental news exposure on citizens' daily lives. *New Media & Society, 24*(3), 760–777.

Green, J., Edgerton, J., Naftel, D., Shoub, K., & Cranmer, S. J. (2020). Elusive consensus: Polarization in elite communication on the COVID-19 pandemic. *Science Advances, 6*(28), eabc2717.

Guess, A. M., Barberá, P., Munzert, S., & Yang, J. (2021). The consequences of online partisan media. *Proceedings of the National Academy of Sciences, 118*(14), e2013464118.

Haim, M., Breuer, J., & Stier, S. (2021). Do news actually "Find Me"? Using digital behavioral data to study the News-Finds-Me phenomenon. *Social Media+ Society, 7*(3), 20563051211033820.

Halon, Y. (2020). Stephanie Grisham: Democrats using coronavirus 'as a tool to politicizethingsandscarepeople.'https://www.foxnews.com/media/stephaniegrisham-callson-dems-to-stop-using-coronavirus-to-scare-public-forpoliticalpoints

Hameleers, M., & Van der Meer, T. G. (2020). Misinformation and polarization in a high-choice media environment: How effective are political fact-checkers? *Communication Research*, *47*(2), 227–250.

Hardy, B. W., & Scheufele, D. A. (2005). Examining differential gains from Internet use: Comparing the moderating role of talk and online interactions. *Journal of Communication*, *55*(1), 71–84.

Hargreaves, I., & Thomas, J. (2002). *New news, old news*. London: Independent Television

Hart, P. S., & Nisbet, E. C. (2012). Boomerang effects in science communication: How motivated reasoning and identity cues amplify opinion polarization about climate mitigation policies. *Communication Research*, *39*(6), 701–723.

Hart, P. S., Chinn, S., & Soroka, S. (2020). Politicization and polarization in COVID-19 news coverage. *Science Communication*, *42*, 679–697.

Hasell, A. (2021). Shared emotion: The social amplification of partisan news on Twitter. *Digital Journalism*, *9*(8), 1085–1102.

Havey, N. F. (2020). Partisan public health: How does political ideology influence support for COVID-19 related misinformation? *Journal of Computational Social Science*, *3*(2), 319–342.

Hayes, A. F. (2018). Partial, conditional, and moderated moderated mediation: Quantification, inference, and interpretation. *Communication Monographs*, *85*(1), 4–40.

Heiss, R., & Matthes, J. (2021). Funny cats and politics: Do humorous context posts impede or foster the elaboration of news posts on social media? *Communication Research*, *48*(1), 100–124.

Hermida, A. (2010). From TV to Twitter: How ambient news became ambient journalism. *Medial/Culture Journal*, *13*(2).

Himelboim, I., Borah, P., Lee, D. K. L., Lee, J. (Janice), Su, Y., Vishnevskaya, A., & Xiao, X. (2023). What do 5G networks, Bill Gates, Agenda 21, and QAnon have in common? Sources, distribution, and characteristics. *New Media & Society*, 1–21.

Hmielowski, J. D., Feldman, L., Myers, T. A., Leiserowitz, A., & Maibach, E. (2014). An attack on science? Media use, trust in scientists, and perceptions of global warming. *Public Understanding of Science*, *23*(7), 866–883.

Hmielowski, J. D., Hutchens, M. J., & Beam, M. A. (2020). Asymmetry of partisan media effects? Examining the reinforcing process of conservative and liberal media with political beliefs. *Political Communication*, *37*(6), 852–868.

Hmielowski, J. D., Staggs, S., Hutchens, M. J., & Beam, M. A. (2022). Talking politics: The relationship between supportive and opposing discussion with partisan media credibility and use. *Communication Research*, *49*(2), 221–244.

Hong, H. (2011). An extension of the extended parallel process model (EPPM) in television health news: The influence of health consciousness on individual message processing and acceptance. *Health Communication*, *26*(4), 343–353.

Hornik, R., Kikut, A., Jesch, E., Woko, C., Siegel, L., & Kim, K. (2021). Association of COVID-19 misinformation with face mask wearing and social distancing in a nationally representative US sample. *Health Communication*, *36*(1), 6–14.

Hornsey, M. J., Finlayson, M., Chatwood, G., & Begeny, C. T. (2020). Donald Trump and vaccination: The effect of political identity, conspiracist ideation and presidential tweets on vaccine hesitancy. *Journal of Experimental Social Psychology*, *88*, 103947.

Hovland, C. I., Janis, I. L., & Kelley, H. H. (1953). *Communication and persuasion: Psychological studies of opinion change.* New Haven, CT: Yale University.

Huang, Y., & Boukes, M. (2022). Does social media keep me alarmed? The effects of expectations surrounding social media attributes and exposure to messages of social (in) stability on substitutive social media news use. *Chinese Journal of Communication, 15*(4), 512–533.

Huber, B., Borah, P., & Gil de Zúñiga, H. (2022). Taking corrective action when exposed to fake news: The role of fake news literacy. *Journal of Media Literacy Education, 14*(2), 1–14.

Ingraham, C. (2020, June 25). New research explores how conservative media misinformation may have intensified the severity of the pandemic. *The Washington Post.* https://www.washingtonpost.com

Iyengar, S., & Hahn, K. S. (2009). Red media, blue media: Evidence of ideological selectivity in media use. *Journal of Communication, 59*(1), 19–39.

Jamieson, K. H., & Albarracine, D. (2020). The relation between media consumption and misinformation at the outset of the SARS-CoV-2 pandemic in the US. *The Harvard Kennedy School Misinformation Review, 1*(2), 1–22.

Jensen, J. D. (2011). Knowledge acquisition following exposure to cancer news articles: A test of the cognitive mediation model. *Journal of Communication, 61*(3), 514–534.

Jost, J. T., Federico, C. M., & Napier, J. L. (2009). Political ideology: Its structure, functions, and elective affinities. *Annual Review of Psychology, 60*, 307–337.

Jost, J. T., van der Linden, S., Panagopoulos, C., & Hardin, C. D. (2018). Ideological asymmetries in conformity, desire for shared reality, and the spread of misinformation. *Current Opinion in Psychology, 23*, 77–83.

Jungkunz, S. (2021). Political polarization during the COVID-19 pandemic. *Frontiers in Political Science, 3*, 622512.

Kaiser, J., Keller, T. R., & Kleinen-von Koenigsloew, K. (2021). Incidental news exposure on Facebook as a social experience: The influence of recommender and media cues on news selection. *Communication Research, 48*(1), 77–99.

Karlsen, R., Beyer, A., & Steen-Johnsen, K. (2020). Do high-choice media environments facilitate news avoidance? A longitudinal study 1997–2016. *Journal of Broadcasting & Electronic Media, 64*(5), 794–814.

Karafillakis, E., & Larson, H. J. (2017). The benefit of the doubt or doubts over benefits? A systematic literature review of perceived risks of vaccines in European populations. *Vaccine, 35*(37), 4840–4850.

Karnowski, V., Kümpel, A. S., Leonhard, L., & Leiner, D. J. (2017). From incidental news exposure to news engagement. How perceptions of the news post and news usage patterns influence engagement with news articles encountered on Facebook. *Computers in Human Behavior, 76*, 42–50.

Kessels, L. T., Ruiter, R. A., Wouters, L., & Jansma, B. M. (2014). Neuroscientific evidence for defensive avoidance of fear appeals. *International Journal of Psychology, 49*(2), 80–88.

Kerr, J. R., & Wilson, M. S. (2018). Changes in perceived scientific consensus shift beliefs about climate change and GM food safety. *PloS one, 13*(7), e0200295.

Kim, Y., & Chen, H. T. (2015). Discussion network heterogeneity matters: Examining a moderated mediation model of social media use and civic engagement. *International Journal of Communication, 9*, 22.

Kim, Y., Chen, H. T., & De Zúñiga, H. G. (2013). Stumbling upon news on the Internet: Effects of incidental news exposure and relative entertainment use on political engagement. *Computers in Human Behavior, 29*(6), 2607–2614.

Kim, J. W., & Kim, E. (2019). Identifying the effect of political rumor diffusion using variations in survey timing. *Quarterly Journal of Political Science, 14*, 293–311.

Knobloch-Westerwick, S., & Meng, J. (2009). Looking the other way: Selective exposure to attitude-consistent and counterattitudinal political information. *Communication Research, 36*(3), 426–448.

Knobloch-Westerwick, S., Carpentier, F. D., Blumhoff, A., & Nickel, N. (2005). Selective exposure effects for positive and negative news: Testing the robustness of the informational utility model. *Journalism & Mass Communication Quarterly, 82*(1), 181–195.

Koc, M., & Barut, E. (2016). Development and validation of new media literacy scale (NMLS) for university students. *Computers in Human Behavior, 63*, 834–843.

Koo, D. M. (2009). The moderating role of locus of control on the links between experiential motives and intention to play online games. *Computers in Human Behavior, 25*(2), 466–474.

Kouzy, R., Abi Jaoude, J., Kraitem, A., El Alam, M. B., Karam, B., Adib, E., ... Baddour, K. (2020). Coronavirus goes viral: Quantifying the COVID-19 misinformation epidemic on Twitter. *Cureus, 12*(3).

Krieger, J. L., & Sarge, M. A. (2013). A serial mediation model of message framing on intentions to receive the human papillomavirus (HPV) vaccine: Revisiting the role of threat and efficacy perceptions. *Health Communication, 28*(1), 5–19.

Kruikemeier, S., & Shehata, A. (2017). News media use and political engagement among adolescents: An analysis of virtuous circles using panel data. *Political Communication, 34*(2), 221–242.

Kuang, K., & Cho, H. (2016). Delivering vaccination messages via interactive channels: Examining the interaction among threat, response efficacy, and interactivity in risk communication. *Journal of Risk Research, 19*(4), 476–495.

Kunda, Z. (1990). The case for motivated reasoning. *Psychological Bulletin, 108*(3), 480–498.

Lata, S., & Nunn, P. (2012). Misperceptions of climate-change risk as barriers to climate-change adaptation: A case study from the Rewa Delta, Fiji. *Climatic Change, 110*(1–2), 169–186.

Lazarus, J. V., Wyka, K., White, T. M., Picchio, C. A., Rabin, K., Ratzan, S. C., ... El-Mohandes, A. (2022). Revisiting COVID-19 vaccine hesitancy around the world using data from 23 countries in 2021. *Nature Communications, 13*(1), 3801.

Lazarus, R. S. (1966). *Psychological stress and the coping process.* New York, NY: McGraw-Hill.

Lazarus, R. S. (1991). *Emotion and adaptation.* New York, NY: Oxford University Press.

Lecheler, S., & de Vreese, C. H. (2017). News media, knowledge, and political interest: Evidence of a dual role from a field experiment. *Journal of Communication, 67*(4), 545–564.

Leding, J. K., & Antonio, L. (2019). Need for cognition and discrepancy detection in the misinformation effect. *Journal of Cognitive Psychology, 31*(4), 409–415.

Lee, F. L., Chan, M. C. M., Chen, H. T., Nielsen, R., & Fletcher, R. (2019). Consumptive news feed curation on social media as proactive personalization: A study of six East Asian markets. *Journalism Studies, 20*(15), 2277–2292.

Lee, J. K., & Choi, J. Kim, C., & Kim, Y. (2014). Social media, network heterogeneity, and opinion polarization. *Journal of Communication, 64*(4), 702–722.

Lee, S., Diehl, T., & Valenzuela, S. (2022). Rethinking the virtuous circle hypothesis on social media: Subjective versus objective knowledge and political participation. *Human Communication Research, 48*(1), 57–87.

Lee, S., Gil de Zúñiga, H., & Munger, K. (2023). Antecedents and consequences of fake news exposure: A two-panel study on how news use and different indicators of fake news exposure affect media trust. *Human Communication Research*, 1–12.

Leeper, T. J., & Slothuus, R. (2014). Political parties, motivated reasoning, and public opinion formation. *Political Psychology*, *35*(51), 129–156.

Levendusky, M. S. (2013). Why do partisan media polarize viewers? *American Journal of Political Science*, *57*(3), 611–623.

Leventhal, H. (1970). Findings and theory in the study of fear communications. In L. Berkowitz (Ed.), *Advances in experimental social psychology* (Vol. 5, pp. 119–186). New York, NY: Academic Press.

Levordashka, A., & Utz, S. (2016). Ambient awareness: From random noise to digital closeness in online social networks. *Computers in Human Behavior*, *60*, 147–154.

Li, J. (2020). Toward a research agenda on political misinformation and corrective information. *Political Communication*, *37*(1), 125–135.

Lins de Holanda Coelho, G., Hanel, H. P. P., Wolf, L. J. (2020). The very efficient assessment of need for cognition: Developing a six-item version. *Assessment*, *27*(8), 1870–1885.

Lodge, M., & Taber, C. S. (2005). The automaticity of affect for political leaders, groups, and issues: An experimental test of the hot cognition hypothesis. *Political Psychology*, *26*(3), 455–482.

Lu, S. (2020). Taming the news feed on Facebook: Understanding consumptive news feed curation through a social cognitive perspective. *Digital Journalism*, *8*(9), 1163–1180.

Luengo, M., & García-Marín, D. (2020). The performance of truth: Politicians, fact-checking journalism, and the struggle to tackle COVID-19 misinformation. *American Journal of Cultural Sociology*, *8*, 405–427.

Maksl, A., Ashley, S., & Craft, S. (2015). Measuring news media literacy. *Journal of Media Literacy Education*, *6*(3), 29–45.

Malik, A., Bashir, F., & Mahmood, K. (2023). Antecedents and consequences of misinformation sharing behavior among adults on social media during COVID-19. *SAGE Open*, *13*(1), 1–14.

Maloney, E. K., Lapinski, M. K., & Witte, K. (2011). Fear appeals and persuasion: A review and update of the extended parallel process model. *Social and Personality Psychology Compass*, *5*(4), 206–219.

Mangold, F., & Bachl, M. (2018). New news media, new opinion leaders? How political opinion leaders navigate the modern high-choice media environment. *Journal of Communication*, *68*(5), 896–919.

Matthes, J., Nanz, A., Stubenvoll, M., & Heiss, R. (2020). Processing news on social media. The political incidental news exposure model (PINE). *Journalism*, *21*(8), 1031–1048.

May, T. (2020). Anti-vaxxers, politicization of science, and the need for trust in pandemic response. *Journal of Health Communication*, *25*(10), 761–763.

McCombs, M. E., & Shaw, D. L. (1972). The agenda-setting function of mass media. *Public Opinion Quarterly*, *36*(2), 176–187.

McKay, D. L., Berkowitz, J. M., Blumberg, J. B., & Goldberg, J. P. (2004). Communicating cardiovascular disease risk due to elevated homocysteine levels: Using the EPPM to develop print materials. *Health Education & Behavior*, *31*(3), 355–371.

McLaren, L. (2012). Immigration and trust in politics in Britain. *British Journal of Political Science*, *42*(1), 163–185.

McLeod, J. M., Kosicki, G. M., & McLeod, D. M. (1994). The expanding boundaries of political communication effects. In J. Bryant & D. Zillman (Eds.), *Media effects: Advances in theory and research* (pp. 123–162). Hillsdale, NJ: Lawrence Erlbaum.

McMahan, S., Witte, K., & Meyer, J. A. (1998). The perception of risk messages regarding electromagnetic fields: Extending the extended parallel process model to an unknown risk. *Health Communication, 10*(3), 247–259.

Meraz, S., & Papacharissi, Z. (2013). Networked gatekeeping and networked framing on# Egypt. *The International Journal of Press/Politics, 18*(2), 138–166.

Merten, L. (2021). Block, hide or follow—personal news curation practices on social media. *Digital Journalism, 9*(8), 1018–1039.

Miller, A. H., & Listhaug, O. (1990). Political parties and confidence in government: A comparison of Norway, Sweden and the United States. *British Journal of Political Science, 20*(3), 357–386.

Miller, J. M., Saunders, K. L., & Farhart, C. E. (2016). Conspiracy endorsement as motivated reasoning: The moderating roles of political knowledge and trust. *American Journal of Political Science, 60*(4), 824–844.

Mitchell, A., Jurkowitz, M., Oliphant, J. B., & Shearer, E. (2021, February 22). *2. Republicans who relied on Trump for news in 2020 diverged from others in GOP in views of COVID-19, election.* Pew Research Center's Journalism Project. https://www.journalism.org/2021/02/22/republicans-who-relied-on-trump-for-news-in-2020-diverged-from-others-in-gop-in-views-of-covid-19-election/

Moon, W. K., Atkinson, L., Kahlor, L. A., Yun, C., & Son, H. (2022). US political partisanship and COVID-19: Risk information seeking and prevention behaviors. *Health Communication, 37*(13), 1671–1681.

Morris, K. (2021). COVID-19 vaccine hesitancy: Misperception, distress, and skepticism. *Review of Contemporary Philosophy,* (20), 105–116.

Motta, M., Stecula, D., & Farhart, C. (2020). How right-leaning media coverage of COVID-19 facilitated the spread of misinformation in the early stages of the pandemic in the US. *Canadian Journal of Political Science/Revue Canadienne de Science Politique, 53*(2), 335–342.

Moxnes, E., & Saysel, A. K. (2009). Misperceptions of global climate change: Information policies. *Climatic Change, 93*(1–2), 15.

Myrick, J. G. (2017). The role of emotions and social cognitive variables in online health information seeking processes and effects. *Computers in Human Behavior, 68*, 422–433.

Nan, X., Dahlstrom, M. F., Richards, A., & Rangarajan, S. (2015). Influence of evidence type and narrative type on HPV risk perception and intention to obtain the HPV vaccine. *Health Communication, 30*(3), 301–308.

Nanz, A., & Matthes, J. (2020). Learning from incidental exposure to political information in online environments. *Journal of Communication, 70*(6), 769–793.

Nechushtai, E., & Lewis, S. C. (2019). What kind of news gatekeepers do we want machines to be? Filter bubbles, fragmentation, and the normative dimensions of algorithmic recommendations. *Computers in Human Behavior, 90*, 298–307.

Newman, N., Fletcher, R., Kalogeropoulos, A., & Nielsen, R. (2019). *Reuters Institute Digital News Report 2019.* Oxford: Reuters Institute for the Study of Journalism. Retrieved from http://www.digitalnewsreport.org/survey/2019

Nyhan, B. (2020). Facts and myths about misperceptions. *Journal of Economic Perspectives, 34*(3), 220–236.

Nyhan, B. (2021). Why the backfire effect does not explain the durability of political misperceptions. *Proceedings of the National Academy of Sciences, 118*(15), e1912440117.

Nyhan, B., & Reifler, J. (2010). When corrections fail: The persistence of political misperceptions. *Political Behavior*, *32*, 303–330.

Palamenghi, L., Barello, S., Boccia, S., & Graffigna, G. (2020). Mistrust in biomedical research and vaccine hesitancy: The forefront challenge in the battle against COVID-19 in Italy. *European Journal of Epidemiology*, *35*, 785–788.

Papacharissi, Z. (2015). Toward new journalism (s) affective news, hybridity, and liminal spaces. *Journalism Studies*, *16*(1), 27–40.

Park, C. S., & Kaye, B. K. (2020). What's this? Incidental exposure to news on social media, news-finds-me perception, news efficacy, and news consumption. *Mass Communication & Society*, *23*(2), 157–180.

Popova, L. (2012). The extended parallel process model: Illuminating the gaps in research. *Health Education & Behavior*, *39*(4), 455–473.

Prior, M. (2005). News vs. entertainment: How increasing media choice widens gaps in political knowledge and turnout. *American Journal of Political Science*, *49*(3), 577–592.

Razak, M. H. A., & Sabarudin, M. A. (2023). The perception of social media usage on the development of democracy in Selangor. *Journal of Communication, Language and Culture*, *3*(1), 57–70.

Roberto, A. J., Zhou, X., & Lu, A. H. (2021). The effects of perceived threat and efficacy on college students' social distancing behavior during the COVID-19 pandemic. *Journal of Health Communication*, *26*(4), 264–271.

Röchert, D., Neubaum, G., Ross, B., & Stieglitz, S. (2022). Caught in a networked collusion? Homogeneity in conspiracy-related discussion networks on YouTube. *Information Systems*, *103*, 1–15.

Rogers, R. W. (1975). A protection motivation theory of fear appeals and attitude change. *Journal of Psychology*, *91*(1), 93–114.

Romer, D., & Jamieson, K. H. (2020). Conspiracy theories as barriers to controlling the spread of COVID-19 in the US. *Social Science & Medicine*, *263*, 113356.

Rovetta, A., & Bhagavathula, A. S. (2020). Global infodemiology of COVID-19: Analysis of Google web searches and Instagram hashtags. *Journal of Medical Internet Research*, *22*(8), e20673.

RTI International. (2020). RTI surveyed 1,000 Americans about awareness, perceptions of COVID-19. Retrieved March 18, 2020, from rti.org/coronavirus-united-states-survey

Rubin, A. M. (1984). Ritualized and instrumental television viewing. *Journal of Communication*, *34*(3), 67–77.

Rubin, A. M. (1993). The effect of locus of control on communication motivation, anxiety, and satisfaction. *Communication Quarterly*, *41*(2), 161–171.

Ruiter, R. A. C., Kok, G., Verplanken, B., & Brug, J. (2001). Evoked fear and effects of appeals on attitudes to performing breast self-examination: An information-processing perspective. *Health Education Research*, *16*(3), 307–319.

Ryan Hatch, A. (2022). The data will not save us: Afropessimism and racial antimatter in the COVID-19 pandemic. *Big Data & Society*, *9*(1), 1–13.

Schäfer, S. (2023). Incidental news exposure in a digital media environment: A scoping review of recent research. *Annals of the International Communication Association*, 1–19.

Schaffner, B. F., & Luks, S. (2018). Misinformation or expressive responding? What an inauguration crowd can tell us about the source of political misinformation in surveys. *Public Opinion Quarterly*, *82*(1), 135–147.

Scheufele, D. A. (2002). Examining differential gains from mass media and their implications for participatory behavior. *Communication Research, 29*(1), 46–65.

Scheufele, D. A., Hardy, B. W., Brossard, D., Waismel-Manor, I. S., & Nisbet, E. (2006). Democracy based on difference: Examining the links between structural heterogeneity, heterogeneity of discussion networks, and democratic citizenship. *Journal of Communication, 56*, 728–753.

Sears, D. O., & Freedman, J. L. (1967). Selective exposure to information: A critical review. *Public Opinion Quarterly, 31*(2), 194–213.

Segado-Boj, F., Dıaz-Campo, J., & Quevedo-Redondo, R. (2019). Influence of the 'news finds me' perception on news sharing and news consumption on social media. *Communication Today, 10*(2), 90–104.

Segado-Boj, F., Díaz-Campo, J., Navarro-Asencio, E., & Remacha-González, L. (2020). Influence of News-Finds-Me Perception on accuracy, factuality and relevance assessment. Case study of news item on climate change. *Revista editerránea de comunicación, 11*(2), 85–103.

Shah, D. V. (2016). Conversation is the soul of democracy: Expression effects, communication mediation, and digital media. *Communication and the Public, 1*(1), 12–18.

Shah, D. V., Cho, J., Nah, S., Gotlieb, M. R., Hwang, H., Lee, N. J., ... McLeod, D. M. (2007). Campaign ads, online messaging, and participation: Extending the communication mediation model. *Journal of Communication, 57*(4), 676–703.

Shah, D. V., McLeod, D. M., Rojas, H., Cho, J., Wagner, M. W., & Friedland, L. A. (2017). Revising the communication mediation model for a new political communication ecology. *Human Communication Research, 43*(4), 491–504.

Shahin, S., Saldaña, M., & Gil de Zuniga, H. (2021). Peripheral elaboration model: The impact of incidental news exposure on political participation. *Journal of Information Technology & Politics, 18*(2), 148–163.

Shahsavari, S., Holur, P., Wang, T., Tangherlini, T. R., & Roychowdhury, V. (2020). Conspiracy in the time of corona: Automatic detection of emerging COVID-19 conspiracy theories in social media and the news. *Journal of Computational Social Science, 3*(2), 279–317.

Shehata, A. (2014). Game frames, issue frames, and mobilization: Disentangling the effects of frame exposure and motivated news attention on political cynicism and engagement. *International Journal of Public Opinion Research, 26*(2), 157–177.

Shehata, A., Hopmann, D. N., Nord, L., & Höijer, J. (2015). Television channel content profiles and differential knowledge growth: A test of the inadvertent learning hypothesis using panel data. *Political Communication, 32*(3), 377–395.

Shen, C., & Gong, H. (2019). Personal ties, group ties and latent ties: Connecting network size to diversity and trust in the mobile social network WeChat. *Asian Journal of Communication, 29*(1), 18–34.

Skocpol, T., & Williamson, V. (2016). *The tea party and the remaking of Republican conservatism*. Oxford University Press.

Smith, G., & Searles, K. (2014). Who let the (attack) dogs out? New evidence for partisan media effects. *Public Opinion Quarterly, 78*(1), 71–99.

Smith, L., Amlôt, R., Weinman, J., Yiend, J., & Rubin, G.J. (2017). A systematic review of factors affecting vaccine uptake in young children. *Vaccine, 35*(45), 6059–6069.

So, J. (2013). A further extension of the extended parallel process model (E-EPPM): Implications of cognitive appraisal theory of emotion and dispositional coping style. *Health Communication, 28*(1), 72–83.

Song, H., Gil de Zúñiga, H., & Boomgaarden, H. G. (2020). Social media news use and political cynicism: Differential pathways through "news finds me" perception. *Mass Communication & Society*, *23*(1), 47–70.

Southwell, B. G., Niederdeppe, J., Cappella, J. N., Gaysynsky, A., Kelley, D. E., Oh, A., ... Chou, W. Y. S. (2019). Misinformation as a misunderstood challenge to public health. *American Journal of Preventive Medicine*, *57*(2), 282–285.

Sotirovic, M., & McLeod, J. M. (2001). Values, communication behavior, and political participation. *Political Communication*, *18*(3), 273–300.

Stephenson, M. T., & Witte, K. (1998). Fear, threat, and perceptions of efficacy from frightening skin cancer messages. *Public Health Reviews*, *26*, 147–174.

Stolberg, S., & Wieland, N. (2020). Study finds 'single largest driver' of coronavirus misinformation: Trump. *The New York Times*. https://www.nytimes.com/2020/09/30/us/politics/trump-coronavirus-misinformation.html

Strauß, N., Huber, B., & Gil de Zúñiga, H. (2020). "Yes, I Saw It–But Didn't Read It..." A cross-country study, exploring relationships between incidental news exposure and news use across platforms. *Digital Journalism*, *8*(9), 1181–1205.

Strauß, N., Huber, B., & Gil de Zúñiga, H. (2021). Structural influences on the News Finds Me perception: Why people believe they don't have to actively seek news anymore. *Social Media+ Society*, *7*(2), 20563051211024966.

Strickland, A. A., Taber, C. S., & Lodge, M. (2011). Motivated reasoning and public opinion. *Journal of Health Politics, Policy and Law*, *36*(6), 935–944.

Stroud, N. J. (2008). Media use and political predispositions: Revisiting the concept of selective exposure. *Political Behavior*, *30*, 341–366.

Stroud, N. J. (2010). Polarization and Partisan Selective Exposure. *Journal of Communication*, *60*, 556–576.

Stubenvoll, M., Heiss, R., & Matthes, J. (2021). Media trust under threat: Antecedents and consequences of misinformation perceptions on social media. *International Journal of Communication*, *15*, 2765–2786.

Su, Y. (2021). It doesn't take a village to fall for misinformation: Social media use, discussion heterogeneity preference, worry of the virus, faith in scientists, and COVID-19-related misinformation beliefs. *Telematics and Informatics*, *58*, 101547.

Su, Y., Hong, X., & Sun, C. (2022). Red media, blue media, and misperceptions: Examining a moderated serial mediation model of partisan media use and COVID-19 misperceptions. *Current Psychology*, 1–16.

Su, Y., Lee, D. K. L., Xiao, X., Li, W., & Shu, W. (2021). Who endorses conspiracy theories? A moderated mediation model of Chinese and international social media use, media skepticism, need for cognition, and COVID-19 conspiracy theory endorsement in China. *Computers in Human Behavior*, *120*, 106760.

Su, Y., & Xiao, X. (2022). Interacting effects of political social media use, political discussion and political trust on civic engagement: Extending the differential gains model. *International Communication Gazette*, *84*(3), 206–226.

Sylvia Chou, W. Y., Gaysynsky, A., & Cappella, J. N. (2020). Where we go from here: Health misinformation on social media. *American Journal of Public Health*, *110*(S3), S273–S275.

Taber, C. S., & Lodge, M. (2006). Motivated skepticism in the evaluation of political beliefs. *American Journal of Political Science*, *50*(3), 755–769.

Takano, M., Ogawa, Y., Taka, F., & Morishita, S. (2021). Effects of incidental brief exposure to news on news knowledge while scrolling through videos. *IEEE Access*, *9*, 37772–37783.

Tewksbury, D., Weaver, A. J., & Maddex, B. D. (2001). Accidentally informed: Incidental news exposure on the World Wide Web. *Journalism & Mass Communication Quarterly, 78*(3), 533–554.

Thrasher, J. F., Swayampakala, K., Borland, R., Nagelhout, G., Yong, H. H., Hammond, D., & Hardin, J. (2016). Influences of self-efficacy, response efficacy, and reactance on responses to cigarette health warnings: A longitudinal study of adult smokers in Australia and Canada. *Health Communication, 31*(12), 1517–1526.

Thompson, S. C., Robbins, T., Payne, R., & Castillo, C. (2011). Message derogation and self-distancing denial: Situational and dispositional influences on the use of denial to protect against a threatening message 1. *Journal of Applied Social Psychology, 41*(12), 2816–2836.

Törnberg, P. (2022). How digital media drive affective polarization through partisan sorting. *Proceedings of the National Academy of Sciences, 119*(42), e2207159119.

Tsfati, Y., & Cappella, J. N. (2003). Do people watch what they do not trust? Exploring the association between news media skepticism and exposure. *Communication Research, 30*(5), 504–529.

Tsfati, Y., & Cappella, J. N. (2005). Why do people watch news they do not trust? The need for cognition as a moderator in the association between news media skepticism and exposure. *Media Psychology, 7*(3), 251–271.

Vafeiadis, M., & Xiao, A. (2021). Fake news: How emotions, involvement, need for cognition and rebuttal evidence (story vs. informational) influence consumer reactions toward a targeted organization. *Public Relations Review, 47*(4), 102088.

Veit, W., Brown, R., & Earp, B. D. (2021). In science we trust? Being honest about the limits of medical research during COVID-19. *The American Journal of Bioethics, 21*(1), 22–24.

Valeriani, A., & Vaccari, C. (2016). Accidental exposure to politics on social media as online participation equalizer in Germany, Italy, and the United Kingdom. *New Media & Society, 18*(9), 1857–1874.

Van Aelst, P., Strömbäck, J., Aalberg, T., Esser, F., De Vreese, C., Matthes, J., ... Stanyer, J. (2017). Political communication in a high-choice media environment: A challenge for democracy? *Annals of the International Communication Association, 41*(1), 3–27.

Weeks, B. E., Menchen-Trevino, E., Calabrese, C., Casas, A., & Wojcieszak, M. (2021). Partisan media, untrustworthy news sites, and political misperceptions. *New Media & Society, 0*(0). https://doi.org/10.1177/14614448211033300

West, J. D., & Bergstrom, C. T. (2021). Misinformation in and about science. *Proceedings of the National Academy of Sciences, 118*(15), e1912444117.

Wieland, M., & Kleinen-von Königslöw, K. (2020). Conceptualizing different forms of news processing following incidental news contact: A triple-path model. *Journalism, 21*(8), 1049–1066.

Williams, A. E. (2012). Trust or bust? Questioning the relationship between media trust and news attention. *Journal of Broadcasting & Electronic Media, 56*(1), 116–131.

Wilson, R., Zaytseva, A., Bocquier, A., Nokri, A., Fressard, L., Chamboredon, P., Carbonaro, C., Bernardi, S., & Verger, P. (2020). Vaccine hesitancy and self-vaccination behaviors among nurses in southeastern France. *Vaccine, 38*(5), 1144–1151.

Witte, K. (1992). Putting the fear back into fear appeals: The extended parallel process model. *Communication Monographs, 59*(4), 329–349.

Witte, K. (1994). Fear control and danger control: A test of the extended parallel process model (EPPM). *Communication Monographs, 61*(2), 113–134.

Witte, K. (1998a). Fear as motivator, fear as inhibitor: Using the extended parallel process model to explain fear appeal successes and failures. In P. Anderson (Ed.), *Handbook of communication and emotion* (pp. 423–450). San Diego, CA: Academic Press.

Witte, K. (1998b). A theoretically based evaluation of HIV/AIDS prevention campaigns along the trans-Africa highway in Kenya. *Journal of Health Communication*, *3*(4), 345–363.

Witte, K., & Allen, M. (2000). A meta-analysis of fear appeals: Implications for effective public health campaigns. *Health Education & Behavior*, *27*(5), 591–615.

Witte, K., Cameron, K. A., McKeon, J. K., & Berkowitz, J. M. (1996). Predicting risk behaviors: Development and validation of a diagnostic scale. *Journal of Health Communication*, *1*(4), 317–341.

World Health Organization. (2020). Rolling updates on coronavirus disease (COVID-19). Retrieved March 15, 2020 from https://www.who.int/emergencies/diseases/novel-coronavirus-2019/events-as-they-happen

Xiao, X., Borah, P., & Su, Y. (2021a). The dangers of blind trust: Examining the interplay among social media news use, misinformation identification, and news trust on conspiracy beliefs. *Public Understanding of Science*, *30*(8), 977–992.

Xiao, X., Su, Y., & Lee, D. K. L. (2021b). Who consumes new media content more wisely? Examining personality factors, SNS use, and new media literacy in the era of misinformation. *Social Media + Society*, *7*(1), 2056305121990635.

Yamamoto, M., & Morey, A. C. (2019). Incidental news exposure on social media: A campaign communication mediation approach. *Social Media+ Society*, *5*(2), 2056305119843619.

Yamamoto, M., & Nah, S. (2018). Mobile information seeking and political participation: A differential gains approach with offline and online discussion attributes. *New Media & Society*, *20*(5), 2070–2090.

Zarocostas, J. (2020). How to fight an infodemic. *The Lancet*, *395*(10225), 676.

Zhang, X., & Zhou, S. (2019). Clicking health risk messages on social media: Moderated mediation paths through perceived threat, perceived efficacy, and fear arousal. *Health Communication*, *34*(11), 1359–1368.

Zhang, X., & Zhou, S. (2020). Sharing health risk messages on social media: Effects of fear appeal message and image promotion. *Cyberpsychology: Journal of Psychosocial Research on Cyberspace*, *14*(2), 4.

Zhang, Y., Chen, F., & Lukito, J. (2023). Network amplification of politicized information and misinformation about COVID-19 by conservative media and partisan influencers on Twitter. *Political Communication*, *40*(1), 24–47.

Zhou, Y., Myrick, J. G., Farrell, E. L., & Cohen, O. (2022). Perceived risk, emotions, and stress in response to COVID-19: The interplay of media use and partisanship. *Risk Analysis*, *00*, 1–15.

Zollo, F., & Quattrociocchi, W. (2018). Misinformation spreading on Facebook. In S. Lehmann & Y. Y. Ahn (Eds.), *Complex spreading phenomena in social systems* (pp. 177–196). Springer.

3 Social Media as a Pandora's Box

This chapter concentrates on social media. Social media utilization not only approaches ubiquity in the society but also intensively affects journalistic practices. Journalists have extensively adopted social media to assist their works. As social media are rising to prominence, some scholars highlighted the unique opportunities they offered, whilst others accentuated the concerns associated with these emerging communication technologies. For instance, Twitter was seen as a double-edged sword for helping journalists to stay on top of breaking news but creating distractions and distorting facts. In sum, scholars are generally optimistic about social media's role in accumulating public opinions, visualizing the powerless, scaling up social movements, and posing challenges to crystalized norms. Of course, concerns about the slactivism in social media activities also appear frequently in the literature. That is given online social actions such as affordance utilization and expression can already satisfy individuals' psychological and moral needs in civic participation, people are no longer willing to engage in traditional forms participation.

However, some other scholars have lamented the nuisance that social media can warp democracy, enabling the rampancy and uproariousness of populism. Specific to the COVID-19 pandemic, social media have played an unignorable role in informing people with health knowledge, mobilizing epidemic prevention, and forming consensus toward many different dimensions of the pandemic. However, one most criticized is, due to the inadequacy of fact-checking mechanisms and the lack of effective gatekeepers, social media have already become a fertile breeding ground upon which disinformation, misinformation, and conspiracy theories have been circulating. This chapter aims at examining the role of social media use in influencing people's perceptions regarding the COVID-19 pandemic.

3.1 Social Media and COVID-19 Misinformation

3.1.1 Social Media News Use

There is a symbiotic relationship between social media and the "infodemic." A large proportion of research has demonstrated how the information dissemination mechanism of social media have facilitated the spread of misinformation,

DOI: 10.4324/9781032625201-4

giving birth to the "post-truth" era and its structural issues. First, the gatekeeping mechanism on social media platforms is vastly different from that of traditional mass media. Lewin coined the term "gatekeeping," arguing that a gatekeeper, a decision maker who has the ability to select, curate, and affect the directionality of information flow, could decide what information should move into a group or individual whereas what information should not (Brown, 1979; DeIuliis, 2015; Shoemaker et al., 2001). In the context of a news media outlet, an editor typically plays the role of gatekeeper, making judgments and decisions upon what content is suitable for publication among various news items. Indeed, the process of gatekeeping could be contingent upon a series of important factors, including the sponsorship of the outlet (McMillan, 1998; Schiller, 1991), the standard on which the evaluation of news value is based (Harcup & O'Neill, 2017), the outlet's ethics and policies, how other media organization set their agendas (e.g., Du, 2013; Lopez-Escobar et al., 1998; Meraz, 2011; Vargo & Guo, 2017; Vonbun et al., 2016), audiences' tastes and expectations, and other societal, cultural, and ideological factors (Su, 2022). For instance, in the United States, scholars have aptly indicated that much of what is disseminated in mainstream, elite media is left leaning in that antiracist activism "naturalizes capitalist domination" (Dixson, 2018, p. 241; Su, 2022). Herman and Chomsky (1988) formulated the five filters of the mass media in the United States, explicating the very determinants of the type of news presented in mass media. The five filters, namely, ownership, advertising, sourcing, flak, and the anti-Communist ideology, can also be considered as core elements in a media control and gatekeeping process.

Regardless of the various standards, filters, and constraints, the role of the gatekeeper of mass media is still dominated by decision-makers within the media organization. However, in the era of social media, there have been significant changes in gatekeepers and the gatekeeping processes, which may even be an ecological level change. First, the instantaneous nature of social media news information makes it impossible to guarantee the authenticity of news prior to its publication, which clearly provides excellent conditions for the emergence of misinformation. Second, ordinary users, opinion leaders, news media, and large organizations all need to relinquish their original control over news information on social media platforms, as the ultimate gatekeeper becomes the platform per se. In other words, although news media has their unique criteria based on which their stories are published, as long as the outlet becomes a specific account on a social media platform, its content would be gatekept by the platform. Schoemaker and Han (2020) have proposed the concept of supra-gatekeepers, suggesting that social media conglomerates are supra-gatekeepers in that they not only "select and publish content from social media users and from the mass media" (p. 224) but also interact with these agents to create a complex gatekeeping mechanism. In summary, the transformation of the gatekeeping system has become one important prerequisite for the widespread dissemination of misinformation.

In addition to the transformation of the gatekeeping mechanism, the changing role of content producers is also a major driving force of social media's contribution to the "post-truth" phenomenon. Specifically, in the era of traditional mass media, media-content producers are professional journalists who are typically well-trained and possess high professional literacy. In addition, news organizations usually have specialized review departments that play a role in verifying information sources. In the social media era, as every individual who has access to mobile devices are endowed with the right to create and publish contents, journalistic professionalism has lost its foundation, and verification of the authenticity of information sources has also become extremely difficult (Dragomir, 2017; Kwanda & Lin, 2020; Waisbord, 2018).

Against this backdrop, social media platforms, compared to traditional mass media, have become a misinformation hub (Xiao et al., 2021). Amid the COVID-19 pandemic, plenty of research has lent robust credence with respect to how social media platforms play in accelerating the circulation of misinformation as well as the significantly positive relationship between social media news use and misperceptions. (Bridgman et al., 2020; Garrett, 2011, 2019; Lewandowsky et al., 2012; Meppelink et al., 2022; Rojecki & Meraz, 2016; Su et al., 2022b). For instance, Garrett (2019) revealed that social media use had a significant effect on misperceptions in presidential elections. Su and associates (2022b) found that social media news use was positively associated with COVID-19 misperceptions largely because of the "lack of gatekeepers, fact-checking mechanisms and adequate legal supervision" (p. 1356). Likewise, Bridgman and associates (2020) also found that social media exposure was positively associated with COVID-19 misperceptions, which in turn tied to lower willingness to abide by the social distancing measures. Moreover, Meppelink and associates (2022) conducted an analysis of a 5-wave panel survey sample and found that the use of Facebook and Instagram led to more misperceptions about the coronavirus, while the use of mass media reduced relevant misperceptions.

In this section, I build upon previous studies and investigate whether social media news use is related to misperceptions with regard to the COVID-19 pandemic. It is worth mentioning that I explore not only the role of general news use on social media but also the effect of COVID-19-related news use on social media. Besides, misperceptions are of various types, some are general conspiracy beliefs while some are specific to certain issues such as the vaccine. During the pandemic, one of the most controversial topics that has given birth to countless conspiracy theories is the effectiveness of the COVID-19 vaccine. Therefore, in this section, I use two dependent variables, COVID-19 vaccine misperceptions and COVID-19 general misperceptions. Juxtaposing my major variables, this section mainly investigates four relationships, namely, (a) the association between social media general news use and COVID-19 vaccine misperceptions, (b) social media general news use and COVID-19 general misperceptions, (c) social media COVID-19 news use and COVID-19 vaccine misperceptions, and (d) social media COVID-19 news use and COVID-19 general misperceptions.

3.1.2 Social Media Affordance Utilization

News engagement oftentimes mediate the effect of news exposure and behaviors. For instance, scholars argued that active and incidental news exposure on social media can both prompt active news engagement (e.g., Gil de

Zúñiga et al., 2021; Oeldorf-Hirsch, 2018; Xiao & Su, 2023). Through offering abundant technological affordances, social media platforms provide their users with plenty of opportunities to engage in news and information and express their opinions and attitudes. These affordances include but are not limited to the functionalities such as liking, commenting, and retweeting. According to Gibson (1979), the term affordance originally denotes the action possibilities that are "available to be taken while using technologies" (Su et al., 2022a, p. 3964). Based on this conceptualization, technological affordance, as Majchrzak et al. (2013) suggested, refers to "the mutuality of actor intentions and technology capabilities that provide the potential for a particular action" (p. 39).

Larsson (2015) indicated three dimensions of technological affordance, namely, acknowledging, interacting, and redistributing. If we map these three dimensions to social media platforms, the dimension of acknowledging would be manifested by liking, which is also regarded as an affordance for expressing endorsement (Borah & Xiao, 2018; Luo et al., 2022; Thai & Wang, 2020); while the dimension of interacting can be reflected in the functionality of commenting; likewise, redistributing is achieved through retweeting (Su et al., 2022a). Technological affordances of social media are usually positively associated with various types of news exposure (Mukerjee & Yang, 2021). Moreover, Merten (2021) aptly indicated that individuals' utilization of affordances such as their sharing and commenting behaviors could determine the extent to which they interact with the contents, which in turn affects what other contents they could further encounter.

In this section, I include affordance utilization as a mediator. In other words, I explore, in addition to the main associations between social media news use and COVID-19-related misperceptions, whether utilizing social media technological affordances such as liking, commenting, and retweeting could mediate these main relationships. In essence, the operationalization of news use on social media does not entail the dimension of user agency, namely, the extent to which social media users engage in the news they are exposed to. Through examining the potentially mediating effect of affordance utilization, I attempt to provide an account as to whether the unique opportunity of news engagement offered by social media platforms could play a role in influencing the relationship between news use and perceptions forming.

3.1.3 Discussion Network Homogeneity

The degree of discussion network homogeneity determines the strength of the social media echo chambers and the extent of the societal harms caused by echo chambers. As mentioned earlier, the algorithm of social media platforms has greatly promoted the formation and solidification of echo chambers. Specifically, the algorithm can realize both user-based collaborative filtering and content-based filtering. As far as the user-level curation is concerned, the algorithm could facilitate the development of homogeneous user networks by constantly recommending to a single user other users that have been identified as having similar characteristics, encouraging them to establish connections with each other. In terms of the content level, by tracking and analyzing users' browsing records, the algorithm recommends homogeneous contents that it deemed as favorable to the users, thereby strengthening the users' path dependence on consuming a certain type of content. These two levels of recommendation mechanisms have significantly facilitated the formation of echo chambers. Through analyzing a panel survey sample, Gil de Zúñiga and associates (2022) found a positive serial relationship between social media news use, algorithm news preference, and political homophily. Namely, social media news use was positively associated with the news-finds-me (NFM) perception, leading to increased preference on algorithmic news, which in turn tied to higher level of political homophily online (See Gil de Zúñiga et al., 2022).

Opposite to heterogeneity, discussion network homogeneity is typically operationalized as an individual's tendency to or frequencies with which they "connect, discuss, and get exposed to politically similar others, as well as to consume attitude-consistent information" (Gil de Zúñiga et al., 2022, p. 581). The operationalization of discussion network homogeneity draws on two lines of research, that is, people's preference to communicate with those with shared values and ideologies (Iyengar, 2012; McPherson et al., 2001), and people's consumption of attitude-congruent news information (Garrett, 2009; Knobloch-Westerwick & Meng, 2009; Stroud, 2008). Recent research combines both lines of literature to construct the measurement of discussion network homogeneity or homophily (e.g., Gil de Zúñiga et al., 2022).

In this section, rather than treating discussion network homogeneity as a dependent variable, I include it as a moderating variable into the models. I attempt to probe whether the extent to which one's discussion network is homogeneous can vary the significance of the main associations and the mediated associations between social media news use and COVID-19-related misperceptions. Based on the literature I reviewed earlier, this chapter entails the following examinations. First, this section examines four main associations: (1) the main association between social media general news use and COVID-19 vaccine misperceptions, (2) the main association between social media general news use and COVID-19 general misperceptions, (3) the main association between social media COVID-19 news use and COVID-19 vaccine misperceptions, and (4) the main association between social media COVID-19 news use and COVID-19 general misperceptions. Besides examinations of these relationships, I investigate the mediating role of social media affordance utilization, thereby constructing four mediation models. Next, I investigate the moderation effect of discussion network homogeneity and both the four main associations and the four mediated associations, constructing another eight moderation models.

3.1.4 Methodology

3.1.4.1 Data Collection

This survey research was administered through a questionnaire on Qualtrics, and the fieldwork as conducted in October 2021 in the United States. I used the Amazon Mechanical Turk to recruit participants. Amazon MTurk has been regarded as an ideal platform to collect more geographically diversified and politically representative data and to offer a credible source of respondents for studies that aim at examining cognitive processes of human beings instead of inferring general population estimates (Amazeen, 2020; Berinsky et al., 2012; Boas et al., 2020). Respondents were individuals resided in the United States at the time the questionnaire was disseminated. Participants were aged 18 or above. Each participant was compensated with 1.1 dollar. Finally, I sampled 1004 respondents. Upon collection of the initial data, I removed incomplete samples and those spent quite limited time to complete the questionnaire, rendering 915 samples. These samples are the final valid samples sent for analysis.

3.1.4.2 Measurements

General news use on social media. Six items were utilized to evaluate general news use on social media platforms. The respondents were asked to indicate the frequencies with which they get news information from "Facebook," "Twitter," "Reddit," "YouTube," "Snapchat," and "other social media platforms" via a 5-point Likert scale (1 = never, 5 = always, M = 3.20, SD = 0.85, α = 0.73).

COVID-19 news use on social media. Four items were used to measure COVID-19 news use on social media platforms. The respondents were asked to indicate the frequencies with which they follow COVID-19 news information from "Facebook," "Twitter," "YouTube," and "other social media platforms" via a 5-point Likert scale (1 = never, 5 = always, M = 3.88, SD = 0.95, α = 0.87).

COVID-19 vaccine misperceptions. Four items were comprised to measure COVID-19 vaccine misperceptions. Specifically, the participants were asked to indicate the extent to which they agree with four statements, "The COVID-19 vaccine cannot protect people against the virus," "The COVID-19 vaccine will alter people's DNAs," "The COVID-19 vaccine will infect people with the coronavirus," and "The COVID-19 vaccine can cause autism and other conditions" via a 5-point Likert scale (1 = never, 5 = always, M = 3.34, SD = 1.44, α = 0.96).

COVID-19 general misperceptions. The measurement of the COVID-19 general misperceptions consists of nine items. Each item was a piece of misinformation or conspiracy theory, and the respondents were asked to indicate the extent to which they agree with each statement on a 5-point Likert scale (1 = strongly disagree, 5 = strongly agree). The statements include "COVID-19 death rates are inflated," "Wearing a mask does not protect you from COVID-19," "5G radiant is the real cause of COVID-19," "Bill Gates intends to implant microchips in people via COVID-19 vaccination," and so forth. It warrants noticing that misinformation and conspiracy theories do not necessarily mean that the message is fake, it highlights that the information per se lacks any scientific evidence and can facilitate the devastation of the "infodemic" (Himelboim et al., 2023). The measurement of this variable reached satisfactory internal reliability (M = 3.47, SD = 1.09, α = 0.95).

Social media affordance utilization. Three items were comprised to measure social media affordance utilization. Specifically, participants were asked to indicate the frequencies with which they "like," "comments," and "retweet" on social media platforms they use via a 5-point Likert scale (1 = never, 5 = always, M = 3.82, SD = 1.14, α = 0.90).

Discussion network homogeneity. Four items were utilized to assess discussion network homogeneity. Specifically, the respondents were asked to indicate the frequencies with which they discuss politics and public affairs online with "people who have similar viewpoints with you," "people who you agree with," "families and relatives," and "friends" via a 5-point Likert scale (1 = never, 5 = always, M = 3.82, SD = 1.08, α = 0.95).

Control variables. In addition, I also added control variables into the models to remove the concern of spurious effects. The respondents were first asked to report their age in numeric form (M = 37.47, SD = 11.07). The respondents' gender was also measured through a dummy variable (44% female, 56% male). The respondent' race was also surveyed (79.5% White, 20.5% non-whites). The respondents' education level was administered by their self-reported educational degrees (*Median* = 5 [Bachelor's degree], SD = .83), monthly income (*Median* = 4 [\$8000-\$10,000], SD = 1.61). Given the fact that the pandemic has been significantly politicized in United States, the respondents' Party ID was controlled. Party ID was measured on a 5-point Likert scale (1 = strong Republican, 5 = strong Democrat; M = 3.29, SD = 1.53). Additionally, the respondents' interests in news and politics were also added as control variables. News interest and political interest were measured by asking the respondents to rate their interests in news and politics in a 5-point Likert scale, respectively (1 = not at all interested, 5 = extremely interested; M_{news} = 3.90, SD_{news} = 1.06; $M_{politics}$ = 3.71, $SD_{politics}$ = 1.07).

3.1.4.3 Analytical Strategy

To investigate the proposed relationships in this section, I perform hierarchical regressions to explore the main associations between (1) general news use on social media and COVID-19 general misperceptions, (2) general news use on social media and COVID-19 vaccine misperceptions, (3) COVID-19 news use on social media and COVID-19 general misperceptions, and (4) COVID-19 news use on social media and COVID-19 vaccine misperceptions. Further, I conduct PROCESS macro model 4 to investigate the mediation effect of social media news engagement on the four main relationships. Moreover, I use PROCESS macro model 1 to explore the moderation effect of discussion network heterogeneity on the four main associations. Finally, PROCESS macro model 14 was used to analyze the four moderated mediation models.

3.1.5 Results

First, I analyzed the main association between general news use on social media and COVID-19 general misperceptions and vaccine misperceptions. As can be seen in Table 3.1, beyond all controls, general news use on social media is positively associated with both COVID-19 vaccine misperceptions ($b = 0.51$, $SE = 0.05$, $p < .001$) and COVID-19 general misperceptions ($b = 0.48$, $SE = 0.04$, $p < .001$), suggesting that consuming general news through social media platforms is a positive predictor of misperceptions regarding COVID-19 and its vaccines.

Next, when it comes to using COVID-19 specific news on social media, Table 3.2 shows that beyond all controls, COVID-19 news use on social media is positively associated with both COVID-19 vaccine misperceptions ($b = 0.46$, $SE = 0.05$, $p < .001$) and COVID-19 general misperceptions ($b = 0.41$, $SE = 0.04$, $p < .001$), implying that consuming COVID-19 specific news through social media platforms is a positive predictor of misperceptions regarding COVID-19 and its vaccines.

Table 3.1 Main effects of social media general news use on COVID-19 vaccine misperceptions and COVID-19 general misperceptions

	COVID-19 Vaccine Misperceptions			COVID-19 General Misperceptions		
Step 1	*B*	*SE*	*t*	*B*	*SE*	*t*
Constant	4.40***	0.36	12.31	4.86***	0.26	18.78
Age	−0.01**	0.004	−3.13	−0.01**	0.003	−2.88
Gender	−0.53***	−0.09	−6.18	−0.43***	0.06	−6.84
Race	−0.26***	0.03	−8.08	−0.25***	0.02	10.49
Education	−0.18**	0.06	−2.91	−0.23***	0.04	−5.18
Monthly income	−0.33***	0.03	11.18	0.27***	0.02	12.89
Party ID	−0.13***	0.03	−4.20	−0.11***	0.02	−5.20
News interest	0.12*	0.06	2.09	−.12**	0.04	2.82
Political interest	0.08	0.06	1.43	0.02	0.04	0.42
R^2	0.24***			0.30***		
Step 2						
Constant	3.04***	0.37	8.31	3.58***	0.25	14.08
Age	−0.01	0.004	−1.61	−0.002	0.003	−0.90
Gender	−0.46***	0.08	−5.57	−0.36***	0.06	−6.22
Race	−0.25***	0.03	−8.003	−0.23***	0.02	−10.81
Education	−0.22***	0.06	−3.80	−0.27***	0.04	−6.65
Monthly income	0.28***	0.03	9.97	0.23***	0.02	11.71
Party ID	−0.11***	0.03	−3.91	−0.10***	0.02	−5.01
News interest	0.08	0.06	1.53	0.08*	0.04	2.18
Political interest	0.04	0.05	0.74	−0.02	0.04	−0.58
General news use on social media	0.51***	0.05	9.97	0.48***	0.04	13.41
R^2	0.32***			0.42***		

Notes: Cell entries (b) are unstandardized betas. SE: Standard error. *$p < .05$, **$p < .01$, ***$p < .001$.

Table 3.2 Main effects of social media COVID-19 news use on COVID-19 vaccine misperceptions and COVID-19 general misperceptions

Step 1	COVID-19 Vaccine Misperceptions			COVID-19 General Misperceptions		
	B	SE	t	B	SE	t
Constant	4.41***	0.36	12.27	4.86***	0.26	18.64
Age	−0.01**	0.004	−3.18	−0.01**	0.003	−2.87
Gender	−0.54***	0.09	−6.22	−0.43***	0.06	−6.81
Race	−0.27***	0.03	−8.19	−0.25***	0.02	−10.70
Education	−0.18**	0.06	−2.88	−0.23***	0.04	−5.13
Monthly income	0.33***	0.03	11.03	0.27***	0.02	12.73
Party ID	−0.12***	0.03	−4.15	−0.11***	0.02	−5.13
News interest	0.12*	0.06	2.08	0.11**	0.04	2.71
Political interest	0.08	0.06	1.47	0.02	0.04	0.54
R^2	0.23***			0.30***		
Step 2						
Constant	3.37***	0.36	9.30	3.93***	0.26	15.32
Age	−0.004	0.004	−1.116	−0.001	0.003	−0.314
Gender	−0.49***	0.08	−5.90	−0.38***	0.06	−6.53
Race	−0.26***	0.03	−8.24	−0.24***	0.02	−11.06
Education	−0.27***	0.06	−4.59	−0.31***	0.04	−7.45
Monthly income	0.27***	0.03	9.28	0.22***	0.02	10.82
Party ID	−0.12***	0.03	−4.18	−0.11***	0.02	−5.29
News interest	0.07	0.06	1.17	0.06	0.04	1.64
Political interest	0.02	0.06	0.41	−0.03	0.04	−0.84
COVID-19 news use on social media	0.46***	0.05	9.06	0.41***	0.04	11.43
R^2	0.30***			0.39***		

Notes: Cell entries (b) are unstandardized betas. SE: Standard error. *$p < .05$, **$p < .01$, ***$p < .001$.

In addition to the main associations, I also investigated the role of discussion network homogeneity in moderating the four main relationships, using PROCESS macro model 1. First and foremost, controlling for all covariates, the result of the 95% bias-corrected confidence intervals from 5,000 bootstrapped samples demonstrated, as can be seen in Table 3.3, that the main association between general news use on social media and COVID-19 vaccine misperceptions was moderated by the respondents' discussion network homogeneity ($b = 0.1164$, *Boot SE* = 0.0396, $t = 2.9350$, $p < .01$, 95% CI = [0.0385, 0.1942]), Figure 3.1 visualizes the interaction effect. As can be seen in Figure 3.1, among those with a higher level of discussion network homogeneity, the relationship between general news use on social media and COVID-19 vaccine misperceptions was stronger (*Effect* = 0.4114, *SE* = 0.0807, $t = 5.0999$, $p < .001$, 95% CI = [0.2531, 0.5697]), compared to those with a moderate (*Effect* = 0.2950, *SE* = 0.0581, $t = 5.0761$, $p < .001$, 95% CI = [0.1810, 0.4091]) or lower level of discussion network homogeneity (*Effect* = 0.1659, *SE* = 0.0599, $t = 2.7700$, $p < .01$, 95% CI = [0.0483, 0.2834]).

Table 3.3 Interaction between general news use on social media with discussion network homogeneity on COVID-19 vaccine misperceptions and COVID-19
general misperceptions

Step 1	COVID-19 Vaccine Misperceptions			COVID-19 General Misperceptions		
	B	SE	95% CI	B	SE	95% CI
Constant	2.89***	0.55	[1.8122, 3.9613]	3.13***	0.36	[2.4240, 3.8392]
Age	−0.004	0.004	[−0.0108, 0.0037]	0.0004	0.003	[−0.0044, 0.0052]
Gender	−0.31***	0.08	[−0.4647, −0.1549]	−0.23***	0.05	[−0.3318, −0.1281]
Race	−0.20***	0.03	[−0.2567, −0.1430]	−0.19***	0.02	[−0.2324, −0.1572]
Education	−0.12*	0.06	[−0.2259, −0.0095]	−0.19***	0.04	[−0.2594, −0.1168]
Monthly income	0.22***	0.03	[0.1699, 0.2757]	0.18***	0.02	[0.1426, 0.2119]
Party ID	−0.09***	0.03	[−0.1443, −0.0391]	−0.09***	0.02	[−0.1207, −0.0515]
News interest	−0.05	0.05	[−0.1571, 0.0474]	−0.03	0.03	[−0.0985, 0.0363]
Political interest	0.05	0.05	[−0.0515, 0.1459]	−0.01	0.03	[−0.0772, 0.0528]
General news use on social media	−0.17	0.15	[−0.4635, 0.1227]	0.03	0.10	[−0.1601, 0.2259]
Discussion network homogeneity	0.16	0.13	[−0.0964, 0.4191]	0.25**	0.09	[0.0771, 0.4156]
General news use on social media × Discussion network homogeneity	0.12**	0.04	[0.0385, 0.1942]	0.06*	0.03	[0.0079, 0.1100]
R^2	0.43***			0.56***		

Notes: Cell entries (b) are unstandardized betas. SE: Standard error. Upper-level confidence
interval and lower-level confidence interval in the brackets. $*p < .05, **p < .01, ***p < .001$.

When it comes to the interaction between general news use and discussion
network homogeneity on COVID-19 general misperceptions, the result of
the 95% bias-corrected confidence intervals from 5,000 bootstrapped samples demonstrated, as can be seen in Table 3.3, that the main association between general news use on social media and COVID-19 general misperceptions
was significantly moderated by the respondents' discussion network homogeneity ($b = 0.0590$, *Boot SE* = 0.0260, $t = 2.2683$, $p < .05$, 95% CI = [0.0079,
0.1100]), Figure 3.2 visualizes the interaction effect. As can be seen in Figure
3.2, among those with a higher level of discussion network homogeneity, the
relationship between general news use on social media and COVID-19 general misperceptions was stronger (*Effect* = 0.3277, *SE* = 0.0527, $t = 6.2170$, $p
< .001$, 95% CI = [0.2243, 0.4312]), compared to those with a moderate

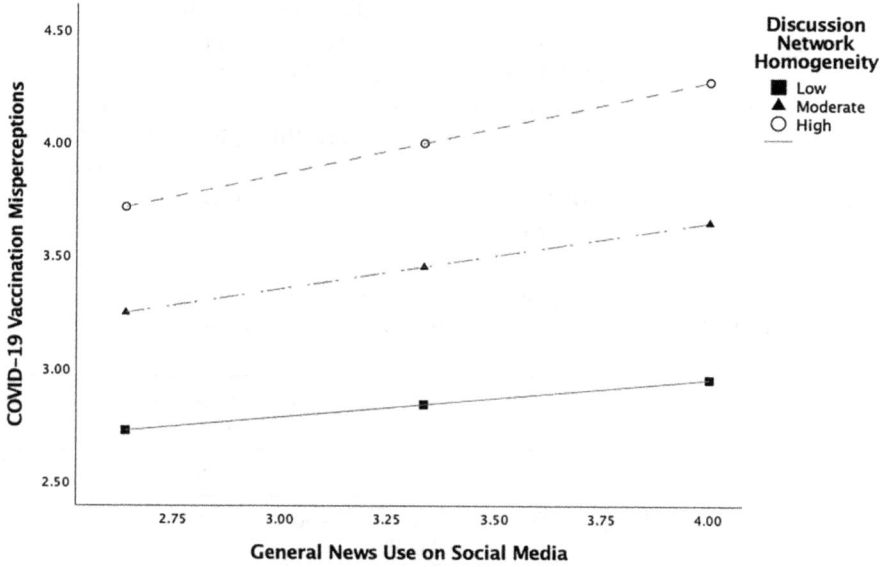

Figure 3.1 Two-way interaction between general news use on social media and discussion network homogeneity on COVID-19 vaccine misperceptions.

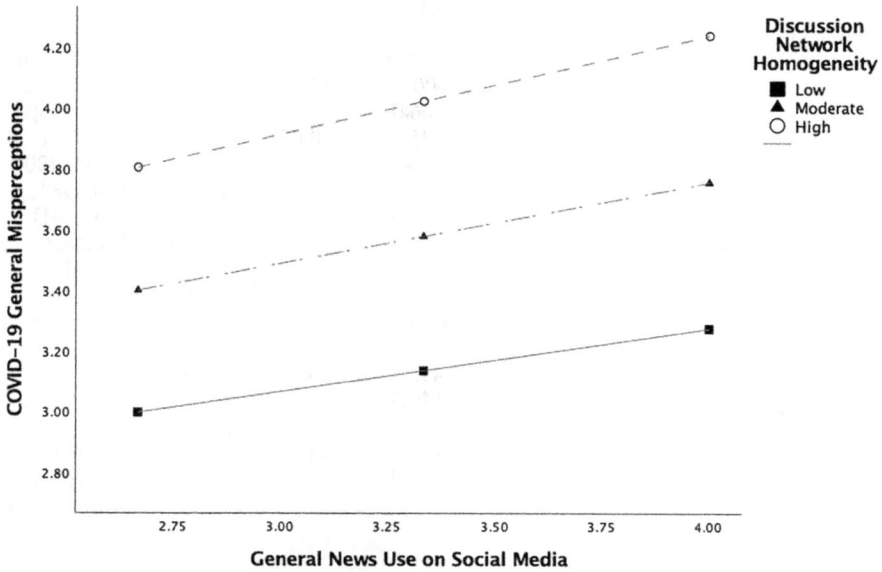

Figure 3.2 Two-way interaction between general news use on social media and discussion network homogeneity on COVID-19 general misperceptions.

(*Effect* = 0.2688, *SE* = 0.0381, *t* = 7.0519, *p* < .001, 95% CI = [0.1940, 0.3436]) or lower level of discussion network homogeneity (*Effect* = 0.2098, *SE* = 0.0384, *t* = 5.4571, *p* < .01, 95% CI = [0.1343, 0.2853]).

Next, I analyze the moderating effect of discussion network homogeneity on the relationship between COVID-19 news use through social media and COVID-19 vaccine misperceptions. According to the output of PROCESS macro model 1, the result of the 95% bias-corrected confidence intervals from 5,000 bootstrapped samples demonstrated, as can be seen in Table 3.4, that the

Table 3.4 Interaction between COVID-19 news use on social media with discussion network homogeneity on COVID-19 vaccine misperceptions and COVID-19 general misperceptions

Step 1	COVID-19 Vaccine Misperceptions			COVID-19 General Misperceptions		
	B	*SE*	*95% CI*	*B*	*SE*	*95% CI*
Constant	3.84***	0.56	[2.7339, 4.9422]	4.00***	0.37	[3.2666, 4.7287]
Age	−0.004***	0.004	[−0.0112, 0.0035]	0.001	0.003	[−0.0043, 0.0055]
Gender	−0.29***	0.08	[−0.4484, −0.1390]	−0.21***	0.05	[−0.3149, −0.1109]
Race	−0.19***	0.03	[−0.2453, −0.1314]	−0.19***	0.02	[−0.2287, −0.1533]
Education	−0.12*	0.06	[−0.2269, −0.0061]	−0.20***	0.04	[−0.2705, −0.1246]
Monthly income	0.21***	0.03	[0.1600, 0.2664]	0.17***	0.02	[0.1335, 0.2034]
Party ID	−0.9***	0.3	[−0.1458, −0.0410]	−0.09***	0.02	[−0.1211, −0.0520]
News interest	−0.05	0.05	[−0.1560, 0.0473]	−0.04	0.03	[−0.1084, 0.0261]
Political interest	0.04	0.05	[−0.0637, 0.1341]	−0.02	0.03	[−0.0850. 0.0457]
COVID-19 news use on social media	−0.36**	0.13	[−0.6142, −0.1114]	−0.16†	0.08	[−0.3300, 0.0030]
Discussion network heterogeneity	−0.16	0.16	[−0.4729, 0.1461]	−0.03	0.10	[−0.2375, 0.1724]
COVID-19 news use on social media × Discussion network homogeneity	0.17***	0.04	[0.1013, 0.2476]	0.12***	0.02	[0.0690, 0.1659]
R^2	0.44***			0.56***		

Notes: Cell entries (b) are unstandardized betas. SE: Standard error. Upper-level confidence interval and lower-level confidence interval in the brackets. † *p* < .10, **p* < .05, ***p* < .01, ****p* < .001.

main association between general news use on social media and COVID-19 general misperceptions was significantly moderated by the respondents' discussion network homogeneity (b = 0.1744, *Boot SE* = 0.0373, t = 4.6787, p < .001, 95% CI = [0.1013, 0.2476]), Figure 3.3 visualizes the interaction effect. As can be seen in Figure 3.3, among those with a higher level of discussion network homogeneity, the relationship between COVID-19 news use on social media and COVID-19 vaccine misperceptions was stronger (*Effect* = 0.5094, *SE* = 0.0867, t = 5.8734, p < .001, 95% CI = [0.3392, 0.6796]), compared to those with a moderate (*Effect* = 0.3350, *SE* = 0.0611, t = 5.4782, p < .001, 95% CI = [0.2149, 0.4550]) or lower level of discussion network homogeneity (*Effect* = 0.1605, *SE* = 0.0523, t = 3.0692, p < .01, 95% CI = [0.0579, 0.2632]).

When it comes to the interaction between COVID-19 news use and discussion network homogeneity on COVID-19 general misperceptions, the result of the 95% bias-corrected confidence intervals from 5,000 bootstrapped samples demonstrated, as can be seen in Table 3.4, that the main association between COVID-19 news use on social media and COVID-19 general misperceptions was significantly moderated by the respondents' discussion network homogeneity (b = 0.1174, *Boot SE* = 0.0247, t = 4.7607, p < .001, 95% CI = [0.0690, 0.1659]), Figure 3.4 visualizes the interaction effect. As can be seen in Figure 3.4, among those with a higher level of discussion network homogeneity, the relationship between general news use on social media and

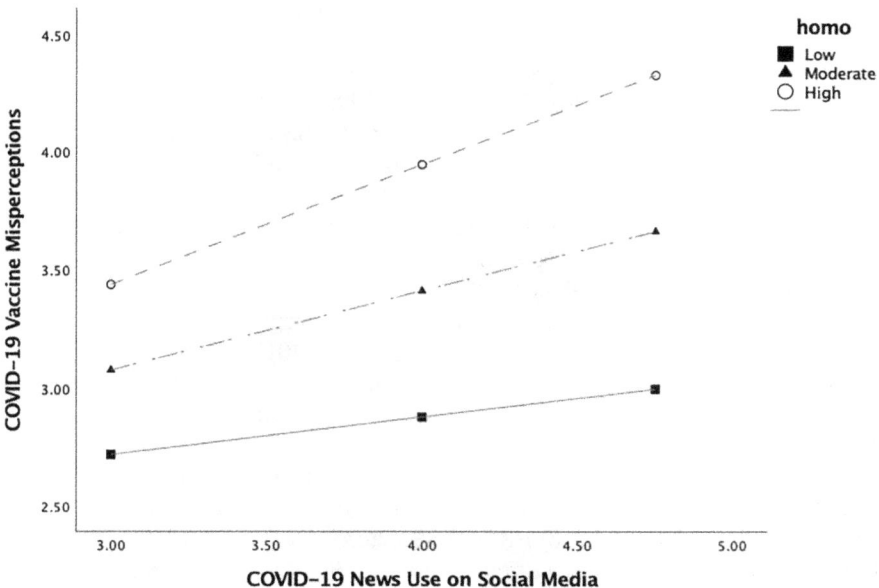

Figure 3.3 Two-way interaction between COVID-19 news use on social media and discussion network homogeneity on COVID-19 vaccine misperceptions.

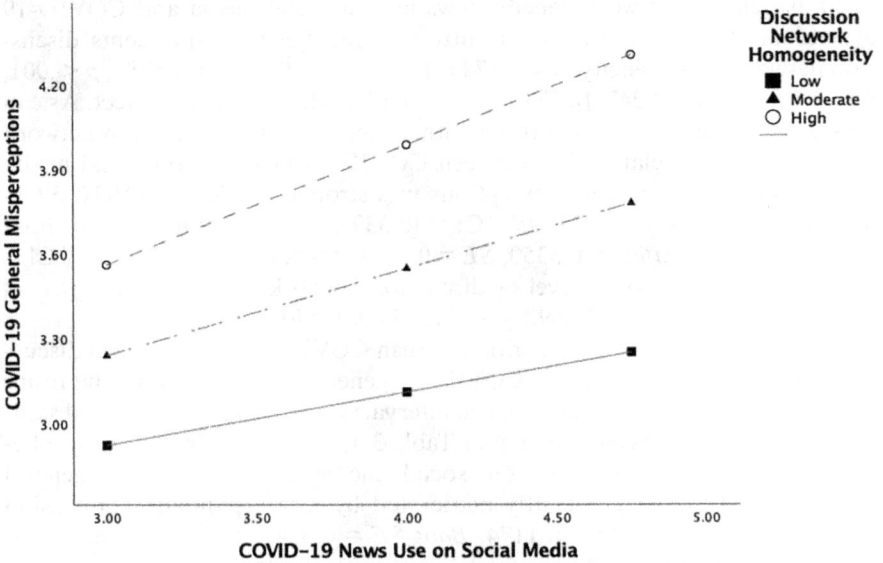

Figure 3.4 Two-way interaction between COVID-19 news use on social media and discussion network homogeneity on COVID-19 general misperceptions.

COVID-19 general misperceptions was stronger (*Effect* = 0.4238, *SE* = 0.0573, t = 7.3896, p < .001, 95% CI = [0.3112, 0.5363]), compared to those with a moderate (*Effect* = 0.3063, *SE* = 0.0404, t = 7.5736, p < .001, 95% CI = [0.2269, 0.3857]) or lower level of discussion network homogeneity (*Effect* = 0.1889, *SE* = 0.0346, t = 5.4515, p < .001, 95% CI = [0.1209, 0.2569]).

Besides the moderation effects, I apply PROCESS macro model 4 to investigate whether social media affordance utilization could mediate the proposed four main relationships. First, in terms of the mediated association between general news use on social media and COVID-19 vaccine misperceptions, the result of the Hayes' (2018) PROCESS macro model 4 showed that the mediation model is significant (*Effect* = 0.1991, *Boot SE* = 0.0265, 95% CI = [0.1496, 0.2530]). Specifically, general news use was positively associated with social media affordance utilization (b = 0.5390, *SE* = 0.0401, t = 13.4556, p < .001, 95% CI = [0.4604, 0.6176]), which in turn tied to greater COVID-19 vaccine misperceptions (b = 0.3694, *SE* = 0.0432, t = 8.5510, p < .001, 95% CI = [0.2846, 0.4542]).

Furthermore, in terms of the indirect path between general news use on social media and COVID-19 general misperceptions via affordance utilization, the result of the Hayes' (2018) PROCESS macro model 4 showed that the mediation model is significant (*Effect* = 0.1202, *Boot SE* = 0.0186, 95% CI = [0.838, 0.1567]). Specifically, general news use on social media was positively associated with social media affordance utilization (b = 0.5390, *SE* = 0.0397, t = 13.5770, p < .001, 95% CI = [0.4611, 0.6169]), which in turn tied to greater

COVID-19 general misperceptions (b = 0.2231, SE = 0.0306, t = 7.2933, $p <$ .001, 95% CI = [0.1630, 0.2831]).

Moreover, when it comes to the relationship between COVID-19 news use on social media and COVID-19 vaccine misperceptions, the results of PROCESS macro model 4 showed that social media affordance utilization was a significant mediator (*Effect* = 0.1804, *Boot SE* = 0.0602, 95% CI = [0.0622, 0.2986]). Specifically, COVID-19 news use on social media was positively associated with social media affordance utilization (b = 0.7083, SE = 0.0350, t = 20.2400, $p <$ .001, 95% CI = [0.6396, 0.7769]), which in turn tied to greater COVID-19 vaccine misperceptions (b = 0.4034, SE = 0.0488, t = 8.2729, $p <$ .001, 95% CI = [0.3077, 0.4991]).

Lastly, in terms of the association between COVID-19 news use on social media and COVID-19 general misperception, the results of PROCESS macro model 4 again exhibited that social media affordance utilization was a significant mediator. (*Effect* = 0.1656, *Boot SE* = 0.0270, 95% CI = [0.1129, 0.2195]). Specifically, COVID-19 news use on social media was positively associated with social media affordance utilization (b = 0.7085, SE = 0.0348, t = 20.3690, $p <$ .001, 95% CI = [0.6403, 0.7768]), which in turn tied to greater COVID-19 general misperceptions (b = 0.2338, SE = 0.0351, t = 6.6581, $p <$ .001, 95% CI = [0.1622, 0.3323]). Indexes of the mediation effects are shown in Table 3.5.

Finally, as I have stated earlier, another goal of this section is to unravel the potential conditional indirect effects of the two independent variables (i.e., social media general news use and social media COVID-19 news use) on the two dependent variables (i.e., COVID-19 vaccine misperceptions and COVID-18 misperceptions) mediated through the social media affordance utilization, the mediating variable. To achieve this goal, I ran four moderated mediation

Table 3.5 Main and mediated associations across general news use on social media, COVID-19 news use social media, social media affordance utilization, COVID-19 vaccine misperceptions, and COVID-19 misperceptions.

Indirect paths	B (SE)	95% CI
General news use on social media → affordance utilization → COVID-19 vaccine misperceptions	0.1991(0.0265)	[0.1486, 0.2530]
General news use on social media → affordance utilization → COVID-19 general misperceptions	0.1202(0.0186)	[0.0838, 0.1567]
COVID-19 news use on social media → affordance utilization → COVID-19 vaccine misperceptions	0.1656(0.0270)	[0.1129, 0.2195]
COVID-19 news use on social media → affordance utilization → COVID-19 general misperceptions	0.2857(0.0342)	[0.2200, 0.3547]

Note: Standardized path coefficients were reported with standard errors in parentheses. INE: incidental news exposure. *p < .05, **p < .01, ***p < .001.

models. The moderated mediation models were analyzed by PROCESS macro model 14, which further demonstrated how discussion network homogeneity vary these indirect effects.

First, the model exhibited that discussion network homogeneity significantly moderated the association between social media general news use and COVID-19 vaccine misperceptions that is mediated through social media affordance utilization (*Moderated mediation index* = 0.0888, *Boot SE* = 0.0191, 95% CI = [0.0524, 0.1267]). Specifically, the bootstrapped 95% bias-corrected confidence intervals suggest that the positive association between social media general news use and COVID-19 vaccine misperceptions mediated through affordance utilization were stronger among those of a higher level of discussion network homogeneity (*b* = 0.2334, *Boot SE* = .0.0419, 95% CI = [0.1521, 0.3191]), compared to those of a moderate (*b* = 0.1446, *Boot SE* = .0.0294, 95% CI = [0.0874, 0.2042]) and a lower level of discussion network homogeneity (*b* = 0.0424, *Boot SE* = 0.0271, 95% CI = [−0.0109, 0.0958]).

Next, when it comes to the conditional indirect effect of social media general news use on COVID-19 general misperceptions, the PROCESS macro model 14 again exhibited a significant moderated mediation model, in which the relationship between general news use via social media and COVID-19 general misperception mediated through social media affordance utilization was varied by the extent of discussion network homogeneity (*Moderated mediation index* = 0.0506, *Boot SE* = 0.0161, 95% CI = [0.0203, 0.0833]). Specifically, the bootstrapped 95% bias-corrected confidence intervals suggest that the positive effect of social media general news use on COVID-19 general misperceptions mediated through affordance utilization were stronger among those with a higher level of discussion network homogeneity (*b* = 0.1141, *Boot SE* = .0.0203, 95% CI = [0.0601, 0.1700]), compared to those with a moderate (*b* = 0.0636, *Boot SE* = .0.0191, 95% CI = [0.0264, 0.1009]) and a lower level of discussion network homogeneity (*b* = 0.0130, *Boot SE* = 0.0220, 95% CI = [−0.0311, 0.0548]).

Furthermore, in terms of the conditional indirect effect of social media COVID-19 news use via COVID-19 vaccine misperceptions, the PROCESS macro model 14 again exhibited a significant moderated mediation model, in which the relationship between COVID-19 news use via social media and COVID-19 vaccine misperception mediated through social media affordance utilization was moderated by discussion network homogeneity (*Moderated mediation index* = 0.1250, *Boot SE* = 0.0252, 95% CI = [0.0765, 0.1747]). Specifically, the bootstrapped 95% bias-corrected confidence intervals suggest that the positive effect of social media COVID-19 news use and COVID-19 vaccine misperceptions mediated through affordance utilization were stronger among those with a higher level of discussion network homogeneity (*b* = 0.3073, *Boot SE* = .0.0510, 95% CI = [0.2077, 0.4085]), compared to those with a moderate (*b* = 0.1823, *Boot SE* = .0.0383, 95% CI = [0.1063, 0.2570]) and a lower level of discussion network homogeneity (*b* = 0.0573, *Boot SE* = 0.0400, 95% CI = [−0.0250, 0.1316]).

Finally, when it comes to the conditional indirect effect of social media COVID-19 news use on COVID-19 general misperceptions, the PROCESS macro model 14 again exhibited a significant moderated mediation model, in which the relationship between COVID-19 news use via social media and COVID-19 general misperception mediated through social media affordance utilization was varied by discussion network homogeneity (*Moderated mediation index* = 0.0787, *Boot SE* = 0.0218, 95% CI = [0.0690, 0.2170]). Specifically, the bootstrapped 95% bias-corrected confidence intervals suggest that the positive effect of social media COVID-19 news use on COVID-19 general misperceptions mediated through social media affordance utilization were stronger among those with a higher level of discussion network homogeneity (b = 0.1429, *Boot SE* = .0.0377, 95% CI = [0.0609, 0.2170]), compared to those with a moderate (b = 0.0643, *Boot SE* = .0.0292, 95% CI = [0.0040, 0.1198]) and a lower level of discussion network homogeneity (b = -0.0144, *Boot SE* = 0.0352, 95% CI = [−0.0860, 0.0540]).

3.1.6 Conclusion and Discussion

Although mass media still haven't lost their grip in agenda setting, emerging communication technologies such as social media have already become the primary venue for most of the U.S. citizens to obtain news (Su et al., 2022b). The glut of information and the transformation of gatekeepers on social media have allowed individuals to easily get misinformed by the various misinformation, disinformation, and conspiracy theories (Allcott et al., 2019; Allington et al., 2021; Apuke & Omar, 2021; Gupta et al., 2020; Himelboim et al., 2023; Xiao et al., 2021). This section analyses a U.S. survey sample and found that using general news and COVID-19 related news on social media were positively related to various COVID-19 misperceptions. This finding is not unexpected as it is congruent with a series of prior research. In addition to these relationships, affordance utilization was found to function as a significant mediator. Specifically, the social media news use could first elicit people's tendency to utilize the technological affordances offered by the platforms, which in turn intensifies people's misperceptions. This finding goes some way to explaining why social media, compared to other news outlets, are more likely to facilitate the dissemination of misinformation. One reason pertains to the fact that social media have offered their users plenty of opportunities to engage in the news production and sharing processes, and it also allows multiple misinformation to spread exponentially simply because users retweeted or clicked "likes" in an effortless fashion.

Among those with a highly homogeneous discussion network, the positive associations between social media news use and misperceptions were stronger. This again confirms the imperativeness to build a heterogeneous online discussion network. Discussions among ideologically and socio-economically homogeneous individuals could prevent deliberation, free flow of diversified information, and social corrections in that people curling up in a relatively comfortable environment are usually reluctant to engage in cognitive elabora-tion as the latter requires greater cognitive efforts (Schwarz et al., 2007). Fur-thermore, the repetitious nature of homogeneous discussions could "interact with individuals' fluency bias, affecting their cognitive processes" (Su et al., 2022b, p. 1365). In other words, the number of times that people hear about a story is positively correlated with their familiarity with the story per se, while with such increased familiarity, people would further spread the story to even more people, creating a vicious cycle (Hasher et al., 1997).

3.2 Social Media Incidental News Exposure

3.2.1 Social Media Incidental News Exposure

Incidental news exposure (INE) could occur in both the traditional media con-text and the social media context. Considering the current ambient news envi-ronment and the penetration of digital devices among the U.S. citizenships, social media INE is more ubiquitous and has indeed received more scholarly attention. (Gottfried & Shearer, 2016; Oeldorf-Hirsch, 2018). As the previous chapter has reviewed, INE denotes a passive news consumption style. More specifically, INE describes a consumption strategy that individuals are exposed to news in an accidental way or just through serendipitous inadvertent expo-sure (Boczkowski et al., 2018). A large proportion of research has been dedi-cated to the examinations of the antecedents (e.g., Ahmadi & Wohn, 2018; Goyanes, 2020; Kaiser et al., 2021; Kligler-Vilenchik et al., 2020) and conse-quences of INE (Feezell, 2018; Karnowski et al., 2017; Kim et al., 2013 Tewks-bury et al., 2001) in the social media age.

Some scholars found that INE can indeed make people well informed about politics and public affairs. Tewksbury et al. (2001) indicated that INE can make people informed as they found from their analysis of survey data that INE to news was positively tied to people's awareness of current affairs infor-mation. Likewise, Feezell (2018) found that INE to political information on Facebook demonstrated an increasing perceived issue saliency. Drawing on a representative survey sample in the U.S., Gil de Zúñiga and associates (2021) suggested that although the main direct effect of INE on political knowledge was not significant or even mildly negative, the relationship became signifi-cantly positive when thorough news engagement and cognitive elaboration were incorporated as mediators in the path. In other words, notwithstanding exposing to news without a pronounced surveillance needs, people can still be well informed politically if they devote sufficient cognitive efforts in processing the accidentally accrued information.

When it comes to the effects of INE on behavioral outcomes, many studies have also shown that INE can facilitate political participation and civic en-gagement. For instance, Kim and associates (2013) revealed a positive relation-ship between INE online and political participation. Specifically, incidentally exposing to news online would probably facilitate people's intention of participating in politics. Similarly, Shahin et al. (2021) found that INE predicted online participation. Juxtaposing this finding with that of Kim and colleagues, it is safe to say that exposing to news incidentally can lead people to engage in both in online and offline political activities. Yamamoto and Morey (2019) analysed a set of two-wave panel data collected before the 2016 U.S. presidential election and found mediated association between INE and both offline and online political participation. In addition to these studies that emphasized the positive impact of INE, there were scholars that expressed pessimistic attitudes such as worries and concerns. For instance, In the context of the COVID-19 pandemic, Borah and associates (2022) found that INE to both mass media and social media was positively associated with general misperceptions and COVID-19-specific misperceptions. Some scholars also dedicated to the investigations of the role of INE through a cross-national lens. Scheffauer and associates (2021) found that network heterogeneity was positively tied to INE in the United Kingdom, whereas "sheer level of political discussion is a positive influence over incidental news exposure in the US" (p. 633).

In this section, I go beyond the effects of social media news use and investigate the relationship between social media INE and COVID-19 misperceptions. The rationale is akin to my investigation of the role of traditional media INE in the last Chapter. In doing so, I attempt to enrich the literature on misperceptions in a public health crisis context.

3.2.2 Methodology

Data used in this section is the same with that of the previous section. Specifically, the survey research was administered through a questionnaire on Qualtrics, and the fieldwork as conducted in October 2021 in the United States. Amazon Mechanical Turk was used for participants recruitment. Respondents were individuals resided within the territory of the United States at the time the questionnaire was circulated. Participants were aged 18 or above. Each participant was compensated with 1.1 dollar. Finally, I sampled 1004 respondents. Upon removal of invalid samples, 915 valid samples were yielded and sent for analysis.

3.2.2.1 Measurements

Social media INE. Three items were used to measure social media INE. Specifically, the respondents were asked to indicate the frequencies with which they unintentionally encounter news from "Facebook," "Twitter," and "other social media" via a 5-point Likert scale (1 = never, 5 = always, $M = 3.78$, $SD = 1.27$, $\alpha = 0.91$).

COVID-19 Vaccine misperceptions. Four items were comprised to measure COVID-19 vaccine misperceptions. Specifically, the participants were asked to indicate the extent to which they agree with five statements, "The COVID-19 vaccine cannot protect people against the virus," "The COVID-19 vaccine will alter people's DNAs," "The COVID-19 vaccine will infect people with the coronavirus," and "The COVID-19 vaccine can cause autism and other conditions" via a 5-point Likert scale (1 = never, 5 = always, $M = 3.34$, $SD = 1.44$, $\alpha = 0.96$).

COVID-19 general misperceptions. The measurement of the COVID-19 general misperceptions consists of nine items. Each item was a piece of misinformation or conspiracy theory, and the respondents were asked to indicate the extent to which they agree with each statement on a 5-point Likert scale (1 = strongly disagree, 5 = strongly agree). The statements include "COVID-19 death rates are inflated," "Wearing a mask does not protect you from COVID-19," "5G radiant is the real cause of COVID-19," "Bill Gates intends to implant microchips in people via COVID-19 vaccination," and so forth. It warrants noticing that misinformation and conspiracy theories do not necessarily mean that the message is fake, it highlights that the information per se lacks any scientific evidence and can facilitate the devastation of the "infodemic" (Himelboim et al., 2023). The measurement of this variable reached satisfactory internal reliability ($M = 3.47$, $SD = 1.09$, $\alpha = 0.95$).

3.2.2.2 Analytical Strategy

I apply hierarchical regression to analyse the following relationships: (a) the relationship between social media INE and COVID-19 vaccine misperceptions, and (b) the relationship between social media INE and COVID-19 general misperceptions.

3.2.3 Results

First, I analyse the main association between social media INE and COVID-19 vaccine misperceptions. As can be seen in Table 3.6, beyond all controls, social media INE was found to be positively associated with COVID-19 vaccine misperceptions ($b = 0.36$, $SE = 0.04$, $p < .001$). Moreover, when it comes to the association between social media INE and COVID-19 general misperceptions, results also demonstrated a significantly positive relationship ($b = 0.30$, $SE = 0.03$, $p < .001$).

3.2.4 Conclusion and Discussion

Incidental news exposure, albeit largely conducive to an informed citizenry, also potentially entails the reinforcement of misperceptions at some point. This section reveals that amidst the COVID-19 pandemic, social media INE was positively associated with COVID-19 general misperceptions and vaccine-related misperceptions. This finding is at odds with a bulk of prior research, which argued that INE and knowledge are positively correlated. However, this inconsistency may precisely be where the contribution of this empirical study lies. Specifically, the role of INE in facilitating learning and knowledge acquisition might be conditional rather than universal. For instance, against the background of the COVID-19, during which an "infodemic" has made people lost a

Table 3.6 Main effects of social media INE on COVID-19 vaccine misperceptions and COVID-19 general misperceptions

Step 1	COVID-19 Vaccine Misperceptions			COVID-19 General Misperceptions		
	B	SE	t	B	SE	t
Constant	4.52***	0.36	12.44	4.95***	0.26	18.73
Age	−0.01**	0.004	−3.26	−0.01**	0.003	−2.98
Gender	−0.55***	0.09	−6.33	−0.43***	0.06	−6.72
Race	−0.27***	0.03	−8.18	−0.25***	0.02	−10.62
Education	−0.21**	0.06	−3.28	−0.26***	0.05	−5.62
Monthly income	0.33***	0.03	11.04	0.28***	0.02	12.80
Party ID	−0.12***	0.03	−4.00	−0.11***	0.02	−4.78
News interest	0.11†	0.06	1.96	0.12**	0.04	2.79
Political interest	0.11†	0.06	1.85	0.03	0.04	0.69
R^2	0.25***			0.31***		
Step 2						
Constant	3.77***	0.36	10.61	4.31***	0.25	17.01
Age	−0.003	0.004	−0.68	−0.000	0.003	−0.02
Gender	−0.51***	0.08	−6.10	−0.39***	0.06	−6.55
Race	−0.26***	0.03	−8.45	−0.25***	0.02	−11.18
Education	−0.29***	0.06	−4.81	−0.33***	0.04	−7.59
Monthly income	0.29***	0.03	10.14	0.25***	0.02	11.98
Party ID	−0.12***	0.03	−4.22	−0.11***	0.02	−5.13
News interest	0.06	0.06	1.03	0.07†	0.04	1.77
Political interest	0.03	0.06	0.62	−0.03	0.04	−0.81
Social media INE	0.36***	0.04	9.49	0.30***	0.03	11.10
R^2	0.32***			0.40***		

Notes: Cell entries (b) are unstandardized betas. SE: Standard error. † $p < .10$, * $p < .05$, ** $p < .01$, *** $p < .001$.

reliable guidance to navigate through the massive amount of information, getting authentic information and knowledge through incidental news exposure without necessary assistance of fact-checking mechanism and media literacy skills could only lead to the crystallization of misperceptions rather than the acquisition of authentic knowledge.

In this case, we should be able to infer that, regardless of people's media literacy, the overall information environment in fact plays a key role in determining whether the societal consequences of INE are positive or negative. More specifically, if the overall information environment is filled with plenty of garbage news, conspiracy theories, misinformation, and disinformation, then INE would undoubtedly result in the strengthening of misperceptions rather than the acquisition of scientific knowledge. However, if the entire information environment of a society is relatively healthy, then such passive news consumption strategy would not necessarily lead to the reinforcement of conspiracy theories endorsement and misbeliefs. This explains why a line of previous research, which was not grounded in a backdrop of social crises or a period of time when misinformation flourishes, has exhibited a positive relationship between INE and knowledge, while the current section and some other COVID-19-based studies (e.g., Borah et al., 2022) found that INE in fact is a significant predictor of misperceptions.

In this way, people's media literacy should be deemed an important internal shield that helps them to become immune to misinformation to a certain extent in this "infodemic" era. That is to say, when the overall media environment is filled with a large amount of misinformation, and social media platforms are still at loss for scientifically and effectively managing the "infodemic," what people could rely on while navigating through the massive amount of information is their media literacy, or say, their ability to identify and discern misinformation, particularly considering that misinformation on social media are usually framed as it looks like authentic information. Although the research results in this Chapter painted a relatively pessimistic picture, I will extend this line of research in the following Chapter and investigate whether media literacy could indeed be a silver lining in preventing people from further falling for misinformation.

References

Ahmadi, M., & Wohn, D. Y. (2018). The antecedents of incidental news exposure on social media. *Social Media+ Society*, *4*(2), 2056305118772827.

Allcott, H., Gentzkow, M., & Yu, C. (2019). Trends in the diffusion of misinformation on social media. *Research & Politics*, *6*(2), 2053168019848554.

Allington, D., Duffy, B., Wessely, S., Dhavan, N., & Rubin, J. (2021). Health-protective behaviour, social media usage and conspiracy belief during the COVID-19 public health emergency. *Psychological Medicine*, *51*(10), 1763–1769.

Amazeen, M. A. (2020). News in an era of content confusion: Effects of news use motivations and context on native advertising and digital news perceptions. *Journalism & Mass Communication Quarterly*, *97*(1), 161–187.

Apuke, O. D., & Omar, B. (2021). Fake news and COVID-19: modelling the predictors of fake news sharing among social media users. *Telematics and Informatics*, *56*, 101475.

Berinsky, A. J., Huber, G. A., & Lenz, G. S. (2012). Evaluating online labor markets for experimental research: Amazon.com's Mechanical Turk. *Political Analysis*, *20*, 351–368.

Boczkowski, P. J., Mitchelstein, E., & Matassi, M. (2018). "News comes across when I'm in a moment of leisure": Understanding the practices of incidental news consumption on social media. *New Media & Society*, *20*(10), 3523–3539.

Boas, T. C., Christenson, D. P., & Glick, D. M. (2020). Recruiting large online samples in the United States and India: Facebook, mechanical turk, and qualtrics. *Political Science Research and Methods*, *8*(2), 232–250.

Borah, P., Su, Y., Xiao, X., & Lee, D. K. L. (2022). Incidental news exposure and COVID-19 misperceptions: A moderated-mediation model. *Computers in Human Behavior*, *129*, 107173.

Borah, P., & Xiao, X. (2018). The importance of 'likes': The interplay of message framing, source, and social endorsement on credibility perceptions of health information on Facebook. *Journal of Health Communication*, *23*(4), 399–411.

Bridgman, A., Merkley, E., Loewen, P. J., Owen, T., Ruths, D., Teichmann, L., & Zhilin, O. (2020). The causes and consequences of COVID-19 misperceptions:

Understanding the role of news and social media. *Harvard Kennedy School (HKS) Misinformation Review.* https://doi.org/10.37016/mr-2020-028

Brown, R. M. (1979). The gatekeeper reassessed: A return to Lewin. *Journalism Quarterly, 56*(3), 595–679.

DeIuliis, D. (2015). Gatekeeping theory from social fields to social networks. *Communication Research Trends, 34*(1), 4–23.

Dixson, A. D. (2018). "What's going on?": A critical race theory perspective on Black Lives Matter and activism in education. *Urban Education, 53*(2), 231–247.

Dragomir, A. M. (2017). The fake news phenomenon in the social media era. *Strategic Impact*, (65), 54–65.

Du, Y. R. (2013). Intermedia agenda-setting in the age of globalization: A multinational agenda-setting test. *Global Media and Communication, 9*(1), 19–36.

Feezell, J. T. (2018). Agenda setting through social media: The importance of incidental news exposure and social filtering in the digital era. *Political Research Quarterly, 71*(2), 482–494.

Garrett, R. K. (2009). Echo chambers online?: Politically motivated selective exposure among Internet news users. *Journal of Computer-Mediated Communication, 14*(2), 265–285.

Garrett, R. K. (2019). Social media's contribution to political misperceptions in US Presidential elections. *PloS one, 14*(3), e0213500.

Garrett, R. K. (2011). Troubling consequences of online political rumoring. *Human Communication Research, 37*, 255–274.

Gibson, J. J. (1979). *The ecological approach to visual perception.* Reading, MA: Houghton Mifflin.

Gil de Zúñiga, H. G., Borah, P., & Goyanes, M. (2021). How do people learn about politics when inadvertently exposed to news? Incidental news paradoxical Direct and indirect effects on political knowledge. *Computers in Human Behavior, 121*, 106803.

Gil de Zúñiga, H., Cheng, Z., & González-González, P. (2022). Effects of the News Finds Me perception on algorithmic news attitudes and social media political homophily. *Journal of Communication, 72*(5), 578–591.

Gottfried, J., & Shearer, J. (2016). News use across social media platforms 2016. Pew Research Center. Retrieved from http://www.journalism.org/files/2016/05/PJ_2016.05.26_social-media-and-news_FINAL-1.pdf

Goyanes, M. (2020). Antecedents of incidental news exposure: the role of media preference, use and trust. *Journalism Practice, 14*(6), 714–729.

Gupta, L., Gasparyan, A. Y., Misra, D. P., Agarwal, V., Zimba, O., & Yessirkepov, M. (2020). Information and misinformation on COVID-19: a cross-sectional survey study. *Journal of Korean Medical Science, 35*(27).

Harcup, T., & O'Neill, D. (2017). What is news? News values revisited (again). *Journalism Studies, 18*(12), 1470–1488.

Hasher, L., Quig, M. B., & May, C. P. (1997). Inhibitory control over no-longer-relevant information: Adult age differences. *Memory & Cognition, 25*(3), 286–295.

Hayes, A. F. (2018). Partial, conditional, and moderated moderated mediation: Quantification, inference, and interpretation. *Communication Monographs, 85*(1), 4–40.

Herman, E., & Chomsky, N. (1988). *Manufacturing Consent: The Political Economy of the Mass Media.* London: Vintage.

Himelboim, I., Borah, P., Lee, D. K. L., Lee, J. (Janice), Su, Y., Vishnevskaya, A., & Xiao, X. (2023). What do 5G networks, Bill Gates, Agenda 21, and QAnon have in common? Sources, distribution, and characteristics. *New Media & Society.*

Iyengar, S. (2012). New directions of agenda-setting research. In *Communication yearbook 11* (pp. 595–602). Routledge.

Kaiser, J., Keller, T. R., & Kleinen-von Königslöw, K. (2021). Incidental news exposure on Facebook as a social experience: The influence of recommender and media cues on news selection. *Communication Research, 48*(1), 77–99.

Karnowski, V., Kümpel, A. S., Leonhard, L., & Leiner, D. J. (2017). From incidental news exposure to news engagement. How perceptions of the news post and news usage patterns influence engagement with news articles encountered on Facebook. *Computers in Human Behavior, 76*, 42–50.

Kim, Y., Chen, H. T., & De Zúñiga, H. G. (2013). Stumbling upon news on the Internet: Effects of incidental news exposure and relative entertainment use on political engagement. *Computers in Human Behavior, 29*(6), 2607–2614.

Kligler-Vilenchik, N., Hermida, A., Valenzuela, S., & Villi, M. (2020). Studying incidental news: Antecedents, dynamics and implications. *Journalism, 21*(8), 1025–1030.

Knobloch-Westerwick, S., & Meng, J. (2009). Looking the other way: Selective exposure to attitude-consistent and counterattitudinal political information. *Communication Research, 36*(3), 426–448.

Kwanda, F. A., & Lin, T. T. (2020). Fake news practices in Indonesian newsrooms during and after the Palu earthquake: A hierarchy-of-influences approach. *Information, Communication & Society, 23*(6), 849–866.

Larsson, A. O. (2015). Comparing to prepare: Suggesting ways to study social media today—and tomorrow. *Social Media + Society, 1*(1), 1–2. https://doi.org/10.1177/2056305115578680

Lewandowsky, S., Ecker, U. K. H., Seifert, C. M., Schwarz, N., & Cook, J. (2012). Misinformation and its correction: Continued influence and successful debiasing. *Psychological Science in the Public Interest, 13*(3), 106–131.

Lopez-Escobar, E., Llamas, J. P., McCombs, M., & Lennon, F. R. (1998). Two levels of agenda setting among advertising and news in the 1995 Spanish elections. *Political Communication, 15*(2), 225–238.

Luo, M., Hancock, J. T., & Markowitz, D. M. (2022). Credibility perceptions and detection accuracy of fake news headlines on social media: Effects of truth-bias and endorsement cues. *Communication Research, 49*(2), 171–195.

Majchrzak, A., Faraj, S., Kane, G. C., & Azad, B. (2013). The contradictory influence of social media affordances on online communal knowledge sharing. *Journal of Computer-Mediated Communication, 19*(1), 38–55.

McMillan, S. J. (1998). Who pays for content? Funding in interactive media. *Journal of Computer-Mediated Communication, 4*(1), JCMC413.

McPherson, M., Smith-Lovin, L., & Cook, J. M. (2001). Birds of a feather: Homophily in social networks. *Annual Review of Sociology, 27*(1), 415–444.

Meppelink, C. S., Bos, L., Boukes, M., & Möller, J. (2022). A Health Crisis in the Age of Misinformation: How Social Media and Mass Media Influenced Misperceptions about COVID-19 and Compliance Behavior. *Journal of Health Communication*, 1–12.

Meraz, S. (2011). Using time series analysis to measure intermedia agenda-setting influence in traditional media and political blog networks. *Journalism & Mass Communication Quarterly, 88*(1), 176–194.

Merten, L. (2021). Block, hide or follow—Personal news curation practices on social media. *Digital Journalism, 9*(8), 1018–1039.

Mukerjee, S., & Yang, T. (2021). Choosing to avoid? A conjoint experimental study to understand selective exposure and avoidance on social media. *Political Communication, 38*(3), 222–240.

Oeldorf-Hirsch, A. (2018). The role of engagement in learning from active and incidental news exposure on social media. *Mass Communication & Society, 21*(2), 225–247.

Rojecki, A., & Meraz, S. (2016). Rumors and factitious informational blends: The role of the web in speculative politics. *New Media & Society, 18*, 25–43.

Schiller, H. I. (1991). Corporate sponsorship: Institutionalized censorship of the cultural realm. *Art Journal, 50*(3), 56–59.

Shahin, S., Saldaña, M., & Gil de Zuniga, H. (2021). Peripheral elaboration model: The impact of incidental news exposure on political participation. *Journal of Information Technology & Politics, 18*(2), 148–163.

Scheffauer, R., Goyanes, M., & De Zúniga, H. G. (2021). Beyond social media news use algorithms: How political discussion and network heterogeneity clarify incidental news exposure. *Online Information Review, 45*(3), 633–650.

Schwarz, N., Sanna, L. J., Skurnik, I., & Yoon, C. (2007). Metacognitive experiences and the intricacies of setting people straight: Implications for debiasing and public information campaigns. *Advances in Experimental Social Psychology, 39*, 127–161.

Shoemaker, P. J., Eichholz, M., Kim, E., & Wrigley, B. (2001). Individual and routine forces in gatekeeping. *Journalism & Mass Communication Quarterly, 78*(2), 233–246.

Stroud, N. J. (2008). Media use and political predispositions: Revisiting the concept of selective exposure. *Political Behavior, 30*(3), 341–366

Su, Y. (2022). Networked agenda flow between elite U.S. newspapers and Twitter: A case study of the 2020 Black Lives Matter movement. *Journalism*, 1–21.

Su, Y., Borah, P., & Xiao, X. (2022b). Understanding the "infodemic": Social media news use, homogeneous online discussion, self-perceived media literacy and misperceptions about COVID-19. *Online Information Review, 46*(7), 1353–1372.

Su, Y., Xiao, X., Borah, P., Hong, X., & Sun, C. (2022a). Consumptive News Feed Curation on Social Media: A Moderated Mediation Model of News Interest, Affordance Utilization, and Friending. *International Journal of Communication, 16*, 3961–3987.

Tewksbury, D., Weaver, A. J., & Maddex, B. D. (2001). Accidentally informed: Incidental news exposure on the World Wide Web. *Journalism & Mass Communication quarterly, 78*(3), 533–554.

Thai, T. D. H., & Wang, T. (2020). Investigating the effect of social endorsement on customer brand relationships by using statistical analysis and fuzzy set qualitative comparative analysis (fsQCA). *Computers in Human Behavior, 113*, 106499.

Vargo, C. J., & Guo, L. (2017). Networks, big data, and intermedia agenda setting: An analysis of traditional, partisan, and emerging online US news. *Journalism & Mass Communication Quarterly, 94*(4), 1031–1055.

Vonbun, R., Königslöw, K. K. V., & Schoenbach, K. (2016). Intermedia agenda-setting in a multimedia news environment. *Journalism, 17*(8), 1054–1073.

Waisbord, S. (2018). Truth is what happens to news: On journalism, fake news, and post-truth. *Journalism studies, 19*(13), 1866–1878.

Xiao, X., Borah, P., & Su, Y. (2021). The dangers of blind trust: Examining the interplay among social media news use, misinformation identification, and news trust on conspiracy beliefs. *Public Understanding of Science, 30*(8), 977–992.

Xiao, X., & Su, Y. (2023). Stumble on information or misinformation? Examining the interplay of incidental news exposure, narcissism, and new media literacy in misinformation engagement. *Internet Research, 33*(3), 1228–1248.

Yamamoto, M., & Morey, A. C. (2019). Incidental news exposure on social media: A campaign communication mediation approach. *Social Media+ Society, 5*(2), 2056305119843619.

4   News Media Literacy as a
Silver Lining

Upon understanding how information sources and news consumption behaviors influence public perceptions and knowledge about the COVID-19 pandemic, this chapter examines the effective approaches to alleviate misperceptions. In this chapter, I endeavor to investigate the role of individuals' news media literacy. Specifically, I explore the effect of news media literacy on different types of misperceptions of COVID-19 as well as factual knowledge of COVID-19. The current chapter also draws upon the survey samples from the U.S. and China, respectively. I argue that the implementation of fact-checking mechanisms by the social media platforms might be worthy of considering, while promoting various types and dimensions of media literacy should be deemed more imperative in this "post-truth" era.

4.1 News Media Literacy

According to the Dictionary of Media Literacy (Silverblatt & Eliceiri, 1997), media literacy is defined as "a critical thinking skill that enables audiences to decipher the information they receive through the channels of mass communications and empowers them to develop independent judgments about media content" (p. 48). This definition has been widely used to conceptualize and contextualize media literacy in a series of subsequent research.

Some other scholars have provided their unique definitions of media literacy, some of which have been impactful. For instance, Livingstone (2004) defines media literacy as "the ability to access, analyze, evaluate, and create messages across a variety of contexts" (Livingstone, 2004, p. 9). By this definition, a four-component model was proposed and has been extensively applied in subsequent research. In Livingstone's (2004) model, access denotes individuals' ability to independently obtain access to certain media outlets and contents. More importantly, such access should be a dynamic process rather than a "one-off active of provision" (Livingstone, 2004, p. 9), in other words, a media-literate individual should have the ability to continually access different types of media.

Of course, from a critical perspective, the extent to which people are able to access media or other technologies are contingent upon their vastly different socio economic status. In the current age of digitalization, this access gap

DOI: 10.4324/9781032625201-5

might have even been exacerbated in that individuals with greater societal, cultural, economic, and semiotic capitals are more likely to accumulate more digital capitals because their inherent capitals are easier to be transformed into digital wealth on social media platforms. For example, a person who had strong social ties and network resources in the traditional era can rely on the popularity of weak ties in the social media platforms to achieve exponential growth in their inherent social ties. In the same way, a person who already has strong embodied cultural capital can also consume more digital cultural products in the digital age, thereby realizing the accelerated growth of their personal embodied cultural capitals. In essence, digital capitalism has given rise to changes in people's way of existence, promoting the dematerialization and digitization of people's activities and forms of labor. Consequently, intellectual labor, emotional labor, technological labor and cyborg labor have emerged. In the competition of digital value, individuals with greater inherent social capital and higher socioeconomic status know better about how to exhibit their uniqueness and give full play to their strengths, and thus become true tide players in the wave of digitalization. Empirical studies have also buttressed this argument. Drawing upon Bourdieu's social capital theory, Calderon Gomez (2021) performed in-depth interviews and concluded that individuals' economic, cultural, and social capitals can all be transformed into digital capitals, whereas economic capital was the most basic form of inequality.

The second component in Livingstone's (2004) model is analysis. The ability to analyze media contents is reflected in a person's understanding of the "agency, categories, technologies, languages, representations, and audiences form media" (Livingstone, 2004, p. 9). More specifically, in addition to being able to access media, a media-literate person should also be able to comprehend the contents of media. In the current multi-media era, multimodal contents have been ubiquitous, hence the "analysis" dimension of the conceptualization of media literacy starts to entail the ability to comprehend media content across different modality (Lotherington & Jenson, 2011; Martín & Tyner, 2012; Talib, 2018; Walsh, 2010).

The third component is evaluation. Livingstone (2004) argued that without evaluation, access and analysis would be meaningless. However, at the same time, one thing to be wary of is that evaluation itself is contingent upon power structure and social class, that is, evaluation standards will vary due to factors such as aesthetic taste, power, and ideology. But these factors that affect standards are closely related to the class attributes of individuals.

The fourth component of the model is content creation. This component is applicable to individuals in the social media age when user-generated content (UGC) has been increasingly influencing the public opinion, the ways in which elite media build their agendas, and even policymaking (Bou-Karroum et al., 2017; Charalambous, 2019; Su, 2022; Weng et al., 2021). In fact, the content-creation dimension of media literacy is rather easily assessed and operationalized. Digital media offers a bulk of technological affordances for their users to create contents and disseminate their products. A media-literate individual is typically able to make themselves visible and create ideal dissemination effects through well-utilizing the technological affordances to exhibit themselves.

Beyond the four-component model formulated by Livingstone (2004), a plethora of other scholars have also dedicated to conceptualizing and categorizing media literacy. For instance, Austin and associates (2021) developed three constructs to operationalize media literacy, namely, media literacy for news sources, media literacy for news content, and science media literacy. Austin et al. (2021) did find nuanced effects across these constructs on both the knowledge of COVID-19 and adoption of behaviors protective for COVID-19. For instance, their findings demonstrated that science media literacy was a positive predictor of COVID-19 knowledge, while media literacy for content of news was not a significant predictor. When it comes to the behavior of adopting the recommended protective measures, all three constructs of media literacy were positive predictors although the effects were mediated through expectancies and willingness.

Park (2012) focused on digital media literacy and suggested that digital media literacy is a multi-dimensional concept. According to Park (2012), the dimensions of access, understand, and create should be corresponded to device and content, respectively. Hence, digital literacy should be reflected in six different aspects. For instance, access to device refers to device ownership, whereas access to content indicates ability to search and filter relevant content. Likewise, understanding device refers to the comprehension of the "basic nature of technology and know how to operate at a functional level" (p. 91), whereas understanding the content denotes the ability to understand and critically analyze content, which is similar to the dimension of analysis in the four-component model formulated by Livingstone (2004). Meanwhile, the dimension of create at the device level concentrates on the ability to create content "using digital technology" (p. 91), while create at the content level refers to the competence to "form opinions, ideas and convert into digital content" as well as "knowledge of the social impact, cyber etiquette and ethics" (p. 91). It is obvious that the dimension of "create" that Park (2012) formulated is an important development and extension of Livingstone's (2004) original four-component model.

Despite the variations of the conceptualization of media literacy, the current chapter focuses on news media literacy, a subset of the broader domain of media literacy (Ashley et al., 2013) and intersects with digital literacy (Maksl et al., 2017). In terms of what news media literacy entails, Ashley and associates (2017) offered a robust model wherein news media literacy contains three vital dimensions, namely, media knowledge structure, need for cognition, and media locus of control. This model, according to Ashley et al. (2017), was formulated based on Maksl et al.'s (2015) news media literacy scale and Potter's (2004) cognitive model of media literacy. In Ashley et al.'s (2017) model, the first dimension, media knowledge structure, assesses people's "knowledge about the institutions that produce news, the way in which the content of the news is produced, and the awareness of possible effects of that content on people." In a nutshell, media knowledge structure concentrates on people's knowledge level regarding news media organizations and their professional routines.

The second dimension, need for cognition (NFC), as I have already discussed in Chapter 2, refers to individuals' preference for processing information using more cognitive efforts. The operationalization of NFC typically entails items that ask people to indicate to what extent they enjoy processing complex rather than simple questions and to what extent they love to have to do a lot of thinking (Cacioppo et al., 1983; Day et al., 2007; Elias & Loomis, 2002; Fleischhauer et al., 2010; Martin et al., 2003). Consistent with a plethora of prior research, my data analyses in Chapter 2 have already illustrated the significant role of NFC in conditioning media effects on people's misperceptions.

The third dimension, according to Ashley et al. (2017), is media locus of control (MLOC), which has also been discussed earlier in Chapter 2. MLOC measures "the degree to which one perceives herself as being in control of whether and how news media influence her." In misinformation research, MLOC was oftentimes used to measure the extent to which people believe that they themselves are to blame if they are misinformed. In essence, if a person is scored high in MLOC, this person is more likely to attribute their encounters and experiences to their own behaviors, rather than the environment or other external factors (Craft et al., 2017; Huber et al., 2022; Nagel, 2022; Su et al., 2022).

In this chapter, I attempt the role of news media literacy in affecting COVID-19-related misperceptions and factual knowledge level about COVID-19. My analysis draws upon a series of recent research. For instance, Su et al. (2022) suggested that although social media utilization was a positive predictor of both general and COVID-19 misperceptions, individuals' self-perceived media literacy was a negative moderator. That is, the positive paths between social media use and misperceptions were weaker among those perceiving themselves as media literate. Borah and associates (2023) also explored the moderating effect of media literacy in the context of the COVID-19 pandemic, they implied that among the U.S. citizens they sampled, liberal-leaning individuals with a higher media literacy for content exhibited lower degree of COVID-19 misperceptions. In this chapter, I adopt Austin et al.'s (2021) measurement of news media literacy and investigate how news media literacy is associated with COVID-19 misperceptions and knowledge in both the U.S. and China.

4.2 Methodology

4.2.1 Sampling

Akin to the previous chapters, the U.S. data used for analysis in this section is the same set with that of the previous two sections. Specifically, the fieldwork of the U.S. survey was performed in October 2021. I recruited survey respondents through Amazon MTurk. The respondents of this survey were individuals that resided in the U.S. at the time the questionnaire was completed, and only those above the age of 18 were recruited in this sampling. Each respondent was compensated with 1.1 dollar. As a result, 1004 individuals took part in the survey. Upon collection of the initial data, I removed incomplete sample, which yielded 915 samples as final valid samples.

When it comes to the Chinese sample, I performed an online survey between November 1st and 15th, 2022, and all participants were recruited through a Chinese crowdsourcing company extensively utilized for survey sampling. The initial raw data comprises 1,465 respondents aged 18 or above who resided in the mainland China. Each respondent was compensated with 15 Chinese Yuan, which is approximately equivalent to US$2.18 based on the exchange rate at the time of data collection. Upon collection of the raw data, data cleaning was proceeded in two steps. In the first step, all the incomplete samples were removed. Next, the crowdsourcing company's website was able to identify the time duration each participant spent on completing the questionnaire. According to Amazeen (2020), samples that spent less than the median time to complete the questionnaire are considered speeders, who might have provided low-quality data. Hence, I further removed samples that spent 18 or fewer minutes (*Median* = 36 mins). Finally, I yielded 1333 valid samples for analysis.

4.2.2 Measurements

4.2.2.1 News Media Literacy

The measurement of news media literacy was inspired by Austin et al. (2021), which comprises two constructs of their literacy measures, namely, media literacy for news sources and media literacy for news content. Specifically, the respondents were asked to indicate the extent to which they agree with eleven statements via a 5-point Likert scale (1 = strongly disagree, 5 = strongly agree): "I think about how someone creates news that I see," "I think about who created the news I am seeing," "I think about what the creator of the news message wants me to think," "I think about what the creator of the news I am seeing is trying to accomplish," "I compare news information from different media sources," "I check to see if the original source of information I see in the news is clearly stated," "I compare new information I see in news with other information I have seen before I accept it as believable," "I look for more information before I believe something I see in news," "It is important to think twice about what news messages say," "I often consider whether a message in news is accurate, and "I check on whether information I see in the news is up to date" (M_{US} = 4.33, SD_{US} = 0.52, α_{US} = 0.72; M_{China} = 3.90, SD_{China} = 0.44, α_{China} = 0.70).

4.2.2.2 COVID-19 Vaccine Misperceptions (The U.S. Sample)

The variable of COVID-19 vaccine misperceptions was assessed by four items. Specifically, the respondents were required to indicate the extent to which they agree with four statements, "The COVID-19 vaccine cannot protect people against the virus," "The COVID-19 vaccine will alter people's DNAs," "The COVID-19 vaccine will infect people with the coronavirus," and "The COVID-19 vaccine can cause autism and other conditions" via a 5-point Likert scale (1 = never, 5 = always, M = 3.34, SD = 1.44, α = 0.96).

4.2.2.3 COVID-19 General Misperceptions (The U.S. Sample)

The variable of COVID-19 general misperceptions was assessed by nine items. Each item was a piece of misinformation or conspiracy theory, and the participants were asked to denote the extent to which they agree with each statement on a 5-point Likert scale (1 = strongly disagree, 5 = strongly agree). The statements include "COVID-19 death rates are inflated," "Wearing a mask does not protect you from COVID-19," "5G radiant is the real cause of COVID-19," "Bill Gates intends to implant microchips in people via COVID-19 vaccination," and so forth. What needs to be reiterated is that misinformation and conspiracy theories do not necessarily mean that the message is fake, it highlights that the information per se lacks scientific evidence and can facilitate the devastation of the "infodemic" (Himelboim et al., 2023). The measurement of this variable reached satisfactory internal reliability ($M = 3.47$, $SD = 1.09$, $\alpha = 0.95$).

4.2.2.4 COVID-19 Knowledge Level (The Chinese Sample)

The measurement of COVID-19 knowledge level was adopted from prior research (Austin et al., 2021), knowledge level of COVID-19 was evaluated with true-or-false statements, with correct answers totaled, based on information from the World Health Organization (2020), the Centers for Disease Control and Prevention (2020), and a contemporary RTI (2020) survey. Respondents were asked to select true or false for the following seven statements: "Antibiotics can be used to treat the COVID-19 virus." "People of all ages can become infected with the COVID-19." "People of all ethnic groups can become infected with the COVID-19." "Eating garlic can lower your chances of getting infected with the COVID-19 virus." "Most people who are infected with COVID-19 virus die from it." "Most people who are infected with the COVID-19 virus recover from it." And "Older adults or those with compromised immune systems are at a higher risk" ($M = .90$, $SE = .16$, $\alpha = .88$).

4.2.2.5 Control Variables

Akin to the above sections, I included control variables into the models to remove the concern of spurious effects. The controls included age ($M_{U.S.} = 37.47$, $SD_{U.S.} = 11.07$; $M_{China} = 37.64$, $SD_{China} = 11.29$), gender (U.S.: 44% female, 56% male; China: female: 55.4%, male: 44.6%), race (79.5% White, 20.5% non-whites), education ($Median_{U.S.} = 5$ [Bachelor's degree], $SD_{U.S.} = 0.83$), monthly income ($Median_{U.S.} = 4$ [\$8000-\$10,000], $SD = 1.61$; $Median_{China} = 3$ [10,0000-30,0000 CNY], $SD_{China} = 1.06$), Party ID (1 = strong Republican, 5 = strong Democrat; $M = 3.29$, $SD = 1.53$), interest in news ($M_{U.S.} = 3.90$, $SD_{U.S.} = 1.06$; $M_{China} = 3.92$, $SD_{China} = 0.81$), and interest in politics ($M_{U.S.} = 3.71$, $SD_{U.S.} = 1.07$; $M_{China} = 3.83$, $SD_{China} = 0.64$). It should be noted that race and Party ID were only used as control variables in the U.S. sample because both factors do not apply in China.

4.2.3 Analytical Strategy

To examine the direct effects of news media literacy on COVID-19 misperceptions (U.S.) and COVID-19 knowledge level (China), I use hierarchical regression and ran analysis through SPSS. Hierarchical regression is particularly valuable when researchers are interested in examining the effects of several predicting variables in a sequential fashion, such that "the relative importance of a predictor may be judged on the basis of how much it adds to the prediction of a criterion, over and above that which can be accounted for by other important predictors" (Petrocelli, 2003, p. 10). Therefore, this analytical strategy is particularly suitable for the analysis of this chapter.

4.3 Results

I first analyzed the U.S. survey sample. Upon running a hierarchical regression model (see Table 4.1), I found that beyond all controls, the relationship between news media literacy and COVID-19 vaccine misperceptions was negative ($b = -0.59$, $SE = 0.09$, $p < 0.001$). Approximately 28% of the variance in COVID-19 vaccine misperceptions was accounted for by the predicting variable ($R^2 = .28$). Likewise, the relationship between news media literacy and COVID-19 general misperceptions was also negative ($b = -0.531$, $SE = 0.062$,

Table 4.1 Main direct effects of news media literacy on COVID-19 vaccine misperceptions and general misperceptions (U.S. data)

	COVID-19 Vaccine Misperceptions			COVID-19 General Misperceptions		
Step 1	*b*	*SE*	*t*	*b*	*SE*	*t*
Constant	4.39***	0.36	12.30	4.83***	0.26	18.70
Age	−0.01**	0.004	−3.10	−0.01**	0.003	−2.81
Gender	−0.53***	0.09	−6.17	−0.42***	0.06	−6.78
Race	−0.27***	0.03	−8.20	−0.25***	0.02	−10.70
Education	−0.18**	0.06	−2.90	−0.23***	0.04	−5.14
Monthly income	0.33***	0.03	11.18	0.27***	0.02	12.86
Party ID	−0.12***	0.03	−4.17	−0.11***	0.02	−5.13
News interest	0.12*	0.06	2.04	0.11**	0.04	2.69
Political interest	0.09	0.06	1.52	0.03	0.04	0.60
R^2	0.24***			0.30***		
Step 2						
Constant	5.48***	0.38	14.28	5.82***	0.27	21.26
Age	−0.01**	0.004	−2.99	−0.01**	0.003	−2.68
Gender	−0.47***	0.09	−5.52	−0.37***	0.06	−6.03
Race	−0.21***	0.03	−6.49	−0.20***	0.02	−8.69
Education	−0.12†	0.60	−1.92	−0.17***	0.04	−3.99
Income	0.31***	0.03	10.66	0.25***	0.02	12.36
Party ID	−0.12***	0.03	−4.07	−0.11***	0.02	−5.06
News interest	0.15**	0.06	2.62	0.14**	0.04	3.47
Political interest	0.13*	0.06	2.29	0.06	0.04	1.56
News media literacy	−0.59***	0.09	−6.77	−0.53***	0.06	−8.58
R^2	0.28***			0.36***		

Notes: Cell entries (b) are unstandardized betas. SE: Standard error. † $p < .10$, *$p < .05$, **$p < .01$, ***$p < .001$.

$p < 0.001$). Approximately 36% of the variance in COVID-19 general misperceptions were accounted for by the predicting variable ($R^2 = .36$).

Next, I analyzed the Chinese survey sample. The hierarchical regression model suggests that beyond all controls (see Table 4.2), news media literacy was positively associated with COVID-19 knowledge ($b = 0.083$, $SE = 0.010$, $p < 0.001$). However, it should be noted that only 9% of the variance in COVID-19 knowledge was accounted for by the predicting variable ($R^2 = .09$), which implies that, albeit positive, the predicting power of media literacy among the Chinese respondents on COVID-19 knowledge was relatively weak.

4.4 Conclusion and Discussion

Findings show that news media literacy is negatively associated with various types of misperceptions about COVID-19 while is positively associated with the factual knowledge of COVID-19. Previous chapters painted a somehow pessimistic picture, unravelling a series of factors that intensify misperceptions. However, analyses in this chapter suggest that news media literacy is a silver lining for effectively coping with the "infodemic."

Misinformation and fake news are oftentimes framed to look like they are authentic, in that misinformation spreaders usually characterize the information

Table 4.2 Main direct effects of news media literacy on COVID-19 knowledge (Chinese data)

	COVID-19 Vaccine Misperceptions		
Step 1	*b*	*SE*	*t*
Constant	0.63***	0.05	13.14
Age	0.001	0.001	0.26
Gender	−0.002	0.01	−0.29
Education	0.03***	0.01	4.53
Monthly income	−0.01†	0.004	−1.93
News interest	0.03***	0.01	3.53
Political interest	0.002	0.01	0.27
R^2	0.03***		
Step 2			
Constant	0.39***	0.05	7.29
Age	0.001	0.001	0.18
Gender	−0.002	0.01	−0.19
Education	0.02***	0.01	3.80
Income	−0.01*	0.004	−2.30
News interest	0.02**	0.01	2.70
Political interest	−0.01	0.01	−0.83
News media literacy	0.08***	0.01	8.71
R^2	0.09***		

Notes: Cell entries (b) are unstandardized betas. SE: Standard error. † $p < .10$, *$p < .05$, **$p < .01$, ***$p < .001$.

with deceptive elements such as fake scientific sources, fabricated quotes, or forgery pictures. The purpose of using these elements is to mislead audience, promote misinformation circulation, accumulate more digital capitals, and achieve certain political or economic goals. Since one crucial component of news media literacy pertains to individuals' abilities to identify misinformation, verify sources in the news that they encounter, and compare different presentations of the same information (Austin et al., 2021), a person scored higher in news media literacy is less prone to fall for misinformation with even misleading elements. Moreover, amid the "infodemic," the identities of misinformation creators and conspiracy theory purveyors are hard to be identified and verified. Since another dimension of news media literacy bears upon individuals' competence to think about what the creator of the news they see is trying to accomplish, those scored higher in news media literacy are more likely to see through the spreaders' hidden plot while less likely to be misled.

Based on these findings, we should be able to infer that news media literacy is imperative in this misinformation era. News media literacy might serve as an internal shield that protect people from falling further for misinformation, disinformation, and conspiracy theories (Vraga & Tully, 2021; Xiao et al., 2021). With the rapid development of information and communication technologies, misinformation will only become more popular and harder to identify, and the "post-truth" phenomenon will only further deepen. Unfortunately, we have yet to see any proven institutional or technological mechanisms being swiftly established and utilized in coping with the rampantly circulated misinformation. In the absence of these external shields (i.e., the institutional and technological mechanisms), the only thing we can rely on is the internal protective shield, news media literacy. We have no reason not to pay attention to the education of news media literacy and media literacy at large. This education should not merely bear upon the simple advertizements by social elites or mass media, rather, education of news media literacy should also become an irreplaceably important part of the K-12 and higher education curricula.

References

Amazeen, M. A. (2020). News in an era of content confusion: Effects of news use motivations and context on native advertising and digital news perceptions. *Journalism & Mass Communication Quarterly*, *97*(1), 161–187.

Ashley, S., Maksl, A., & Craft, S. (2013). Developing a news media literacy scale. *Journalism & Mass Communication Educator*, *68*(1), 7–21.

Ashley, S., Maksl, A., & Craft, S. (2017). News media literacy and political engagement: What's the connection? *Journal of Media Literacy Education*, *9*(1), 79–98.

Austin, E. W., Borah, P., & Domgaard, S. (2021). COVID-19 disinformation and political engagement among communities of color: The role of media literacy. *Harvard Kennedy School (HKS) Misinformation Review*. https://doi.org/10.37016/mr-2020-58

Borah, P., Austin, E., & Su, Y. (2023). Injecting disinfectants to kill the virus: Media literacy, information gathering sources, and the moderating role of political ideology on misperceptions about COVID-19. *Mass Communication & Society*, *26*(4), 566–592.

Bou-Karroum, L., El-Jardali, F., Hemadi, N., Faraj, Y., Ojha, U., Shahrour, M., ... Akl, E. A. (2017). Using media to impact health policy-making: An integrative systematic review. *Implementation Science, 12*(1), 1–14.

Cacioppo, J. T., Petty, R. E., & Morris, K. J. (1983). Effects of need for cognition on message evaluation, recall, and persuasion. *Journal of Personality & Social Psychology, 45*(4), 805.

Calderon Gomez, D. (2021). The third digital divide and Bourdieu: Bidirectional conversion of economic, cultural, and social capital to (and from) digital capital among young people in Madrid. *New Media & Society, 23*(9), 2534–2553.

Centers for Disease Control and Prevention (2020). Symptoms of coronavirus. Retrieved from March 13, 2020. https://www.cdc.gov/coronavirus/2019-ncov/symptoms-testing/symptoms.html

Charalambous, A. (2019). Social media and health policy. *Asia-Pacific Journal of Oncology Nursing, 6*(1), 24–27.

Craft, S., Ashley, S., & Maksl, A. (2017). News media literacy and conspiracy theory endorsement. *Communication and the Public, 2*(4), 388–401.

Day, E. A., Espejo, J., Kowollik, V., Boatman, P. R., & McEntire, L. E. (2007). Modeling the links between need for cognition and the acquisition of a complex skill. *Personality and Individual Differences, 42*(2), 201–212.

Elias, S. M., & Loomis, R. J. (2002). Utilizing need for cognition and perceived self-efficacy to predict academic performance 1. *Journal of Applied Social Psychology, 32*(8), 1687–1702.

Fleischhauer, M., Enge, S., Brocke, B., Ullrich, J., Strobel, A., & Strobel, A. (2010). Same or different? Clarifying the relationship of need for cognition to personality and intelligence. *Personality and Social Psychology Bulletin, 36*(1), 82–96.

Himelboim, I., Borah, P., Lee, D. K. L., Lee, J. (Janice), Su, Y., Vishnevskaya, A., & Xiao, X. (2023). What do 5G networks, Bill Gates, Agenda 21, and QAnon have in common? Sources, distribution, and characteristics. *New Media & Society*, 1–21.

Huber, B., Borah, P., & Gil de Zúñiga, H. (2022). Taking corrective action when exposed to fake news: The role of fake news literacy. *Journal of Media Literacy Education, 14*(2), 1–14.

Livingstone, S. (2004). What is media literacy? *Intermedia, 32*(3), 18–20.

Lotherington, H., & Jenson, J. (2011). Teaching multimodal and digital literacy in L2 settings: New literacies, new basics, new pedagogies. *Annual Review of Applied Linguistics, 31*, 226–246.

Maksl, A., Ashley, S., & Craft, S. (2015). Measuring news media literacy. *Journal of Media Literacy Education, 6*(3), 29–45.

Maksl, A., Craft, S., Ashley, S., & Miller, D. (2017). The usefulness of a news media literacy measure in evaluating a news literacy curriculum. *Journalism & Mass Communication Educator, 72*(2), 228–241.

Martin, B. A., Lang, B., Wong, S., & Martin, B. A. (2003). Conclusion explicitness in advertising: The moderating role of need for cognition (NFC) and argument quality (AQ) on persuasion. *Journal of Advertising, 32*(4), 57–66.

Martín, A. G., & Tyner, K. (2012). Media education, media literacy and digital competence. *Comunicar. Media Education Research Journal, 20*(1), 1–8.

Nagel, T. W. (2022). Measuring fake news acumen using a news media literacy instrument. *Journal of Media Literacy Education, 14*(1), 29–42.

Park, S. (2012). Dimensions of digital media literacy and the relationship with social exclusion. *Media International Australia, 142*(1), 87–100.

Petrocelli, J. V. (2003). Hierarchical multiple regression in counseling research: Common problems and possible remedies. *Measurement and Evaluation in Counseling and Development, 36*(1), 9–22.

RTI International. (2020). RTI surveyed 1,000 Americans about awareness, perceptions of COVID-19. Retrieved March 18, 2020, from: rti.org/coronavirus-united-states-survey

Silverblatt, A., & Eliceiri, E. M. (1997). *Dictionary of media literacy*. Westport, CT: Greenwood Publishing

Su, Y. (2022). Networked agenda flow between elite US newspapers and Twitter: A case study of the 2020 Black Lives Matter movement. *Journalism*, 1–21.

Su, Y., Lee, D. K. L., & Xiao, X. (2022). "I enjoy thinking critically, and I'm in control": Examining the influences of media literacy factors on misperceptions amidst the COVID-19 infodemic. *Computers in Human Behavior, 128*, 107111.

Su, Y., Borah, P. and Xiao, X. (2022). Understanding the "infodemic": Social media news use, homogeneous online discussion, self-perceived media literacy and misperceptions about COVID-19. *Online Information Review, 46*(7), 1353–1372.

Talib, S. (2018). Social media pedagogy: Applying an interdisciplinary approach to teach multimodal critical digital literacy. *E-learning and Digital Media, 15*(2), 55–66.

Vraga, E. K., & Tully, M. (2021). News literacy, social media behaviors, and skepticism toward information on social media. *Information, Communication & Society, 24*(2), 150–166.

Walsh, M. (2010). Multimodal literacy: What does it mean for classroom practice? *Australian Journal of Language and Literacy, The, 33*(3), 211–239.

Weng, S., Schwarz, G., Schwarz, S., & Hardy, B. (2021). A framework for government response to social media participation in public policy making: Evidence from China. *International Journal of Public Administration, 44*(16), 1424–1434.

World Health Organization. (2020). Rolling updates on coronavirus disease (COVID-19). Retrieved March 15, 2020 from https://www.who.int/emergencies/diseases/novel-coronavirus-2019/events-as-they-happen

Xiao, X., Borah, P., & Su, Y. (2021). The dangers of blind trust: Examining the interplay among social media news use, misinformation identification, and news trust on conspiracy beliefs. *Public Understanding of Science, 30*(8), 977–992.

5 Concluding Remarks

With the revolution of the communication technologies, the deepening of postmodernism, and the consistent decline in the public's trust in authorities and the scientific community, concerns regarding the proliferation of false, unverified, and misleading information have been growing exponentially. The concept of "post-truth" has swiftly obtained worldwide attention, and the Oxford Dictionaries named it as 2016's word of the year. In the "post-truth" era, people are no longer interested in exploring objective facts, instead, they curl up in echo chambers and constantly resonate with like-minded others. Consequently, some controversial issues related to politics, health, and science can no longer be effectively addressed, in that the credibility of authority and experts has been fundamentally challenged.

Postmodernism encourages increased individualism and self-enlargement, advocating for alleged democratization and the emancipation of the right to define truth and create knowledge. With the empowerment of the emerging communication technologies, the driving force for people to subvert authoritative narratives and define the objective world all by themselves has been fully activated. Although the "post-truth" phenomenon seemed to have achieved the democratization of knowledge production and the decentralization of information circulation to a certain extent, conspiracy theories and misinformation have also prevailed, severely eroding the existing social systems.

As one of the most significant public health crises in modern history, the COVID-19 pandemic has provided a novel context for post-truth research. Amidst the pandemic, Tedros Adhanom Ghebreyesus, the director-general of World Health Organization, aptly argued that "We're not just fighting a pandemic; we're fighting an infodemic." An "infodemic" denotes an overabundance of information, some verified and some not, that makes it difficult for individuals to find reliable guidance to navigate the current status. Indeed, upon the outbreak of the COVID-19 pandemic, scholars of a variety of disciplines have dedicated themselves to the investigations of the antecedents and consequences of the "infodemic," attempting to point the way to fundamentally address the problem. However, existing literature on both "post-truth" and "infodemic," notwithstanding growing rapidly, has not lent sufficient

DOI: 10.4324/9781032625201-6

credence to their antecedents and ramifications yet, nor has it provided constructive or systematic recommendations to alleviate these issues.

Against this backdrop, this book (1) systematically conceptualizes the "post-truth" phenomenon through identifying its major characteristics and driving forces, (2) examines the nuanced effects of the utilization of different information sources, the passive news consumption perceptions, and incidental exposure to news on the COVID-19 relevant misperceptions and factual knowledge, (3) explores the role of social media news use in shaping misperceptions and knowledge, and (4) investigates the role news media literacy could play in the formation of the COVID-19 related misperceptions.

In Chapter 1, I argue that in a "post-truth" era, the attempts to explore facts and truths are giving way to the resonance of like-minded ideas in online spheres. Moreover, I identify three major driving forces of the "post-truth" era, namely, the technological empowerment, the deepening of postmodernism, and the long-standing public disaffection with the political institutions and the science community. I argue that the combined force of these three factors has accelerated the arrival of the "post truth" era, and particularly fueled the formation of the "infodemic." But at the same time, I also emphasize that the "post-truth" state is irreversible due to the linear directionality of technological development. That being said, this is not a pessimistic point of view. On the contrary, we should consider the current "post-truth" state we are experiencing as a necessary part of the painful process of information democratization. Hence, what is more constructive is to think about how to develop critical thinking abilities to effectively navigate this "post-truth" era.

In Chapter 2, I continue the discussion of the "post-truth" phenomenon while concentrating more on it's antecedents. To this end, I examined the role of partisan media use, incidental exposure to news through traditional media outlets, and people's ambient awareness in shaping misperceptions or factual knowledge regarding the COVID-19. Chapter 2 first reveals that amid the pandemic, consuming two partisan media, Fox News and MSNBC, had significant positive effects on misperceptions. Findings also suggest that people's political ideology was a significant moderator, such that the effects of using both partisan outlets on misperceptions became stronger among those liberal-identifying groups. Additionally, the need for cognition did not moderate the effect of Fox News use on misperceptions, while the association between MSNBC use and misperceptions was moderated by it. In other words, among those with a higher extent of preference for cognitive, logical, and statistical information processing strategy, the positive effect of MSNBC use on misperceptions became relatively weaker. Similarly, trust in scientists also moderated the effects of using both partisan media outlets. That is, the positive effects were found to become weaker among those with a higher extent of trust in scientists amid the COVID-19 pandemic.

In addition, I take a step further to explore the mediating role of message derogation. Findings suggest that message derogation did mediate the positive relationships between using both partisan media and misperceptions. This finding implies that partisan media facilitate people's misperceptions largely through changing their attitudes toward nonpartisan information and sources. In other words, by providing spun and slanted narratives and depictions, partisan media first fosters a derogatory, distrustful attitude of their viewers toward contents on other mass media, which in turn leads to their credulity of misinformation. Next, I borrowed the idea of the Extended Parallel Process Model, revealing a serially mediating mechanism from partisan media use toward misperceptions through the EPPM factors.

In addition to the effects of news source and outlets one uses, I examine the role of incidental news exposure in shaping misperceptions. Although incidental news exposure has already become a truism in the communication literature, most of the extant literature has mainly focused on whether this passive information consumptive style could influence civic engagement or political participation. Few studies have endeavored to address the relationship between incidental news exposure and people's misperceptions regarding major public health crises. However, I argue that this relationship is particularly worth exploring in that the COVID-19 pandemic has become an overriding issue for a few years and has caused lingering impacts. Findings show that incidental news exposure was positively associated with COVID-19-related misperceptions while it was negatively associated with the factual knowledge about COVID-19. Prior studies demonstrated that incidental news exposure can sometimes make people well informed of political issues or public affairs, while here in Chapter 2, incidental news exposure amid the COVID-19 pandemic did not make people truly informed.

In addition to the main relationships between incidental news exposure and misperceptions and between incidental news exposure and factual knowledge, the conditional and indirect mechanisms are equally worthy of attention. In the analysis of the U.S. sample, the significant mediating effect of defensive avoidance bolstered my previous argument in regard to the fact that incidental exposure may lead to avoidance instead of further involvement of news or cognitive elaboration of information. When it comes to media locus of control, findings also showed that in the U.S., the more people perceive themselves as having a good control over their information environment, the more likely they are to be influenced by incidental news exposure to have greater misperceptions. While in China, similarly significant moderation effect of media locus of control emerged in the main relationship between incidental news exposure to TV and COVID-19 knowledge.

Besides, findings in Chapter 2 also illustrate the significant moderating role of discussion network heterogeneity. However, contrary to previous studies, my analysis shows that among those of a higher level of discussion network heterogeneity, the positive effect of incidental news exposure on misperceptions became stronger. This is likely because discussion network heterogeneity may not always serve as an endogenous variable in that it is in fact quite difficult for people to independently choose and curate their own social networks. In other words, even if a person is in a highly heterogeneous social network, it does not always mean that he or she enjoys frequent exposure to diversified viewpoints or discussions with individuals of different socio-economic status and social classes.

Incidental news exposure describes a particular way of news consumption, while the "news-finds-me" is more a perception that people hold in navigating the ambient news environment. Therefore, In the remaining section of Chapter 2, I take a step further and examine the effects of the "news-finds-me" perception of the misperceptions and factual knowledge about the COVID-19. My findings illustrate that the "news-finds-me" perception was positively associated with COVID-19 misperceptions and was negatively associated with COVID-19 knowledge. It can be inferred that such passivity is indeed detrimental to the understanding of public affairs and may even provide a basis upon which misinformation circulates swiftly and rampantly. Moreover, political interest was found a significant moderator in the U.S. context, whereas it did not moderate the main relationship in the Chinese context.

The analyses in Chapter 3 focus on the role of social media news use in shaping misperceptions and factual knowledge about the COVID-19. First, findings implied that among the U.S. citizens, using general news and COVID-19 related news on social media were both positively tied to general misperceptions about the COVID-19. In addition to these significant main relationships, affordance utilization was found to function as a significant positive mediator. That is, using news through social media platforms could first elicit people's tendency to utilize the technological affordances offered by the outlets, which in turn intensifies their misperceptions. Furthermore, findings suggest that among people with a highly homogeneous discussion network, the positive associations between social media news use and misperceptions became stronger. This reaffirmed the imperativeness of building a heterogeneous online discussion network. Further, the relationship between incidental news exposure to social media and misperceptions were also analyzed. The analysis revealed that amid the pandemic, incidental exposure to the news on social media was positively associated with COVID-19 general misperceptions and vaccine-related misperceptions.

In Chapter 4, I analyze the associations between news media literacy and misperceptions and knowledge of COVID-19. Findings show that news media literacy was negatively related to misperceptions about COVID-19 while positively related to factual knowledge of COVID-19. Previous chapters painted an overall pessimistic picture, unravelling a series of factors that intensify misperceptions. However, analyses in this chapter implied that news media literacy might be a silver lining for effectively coping with the "infodemic."

Integrating the findings in the above chapters, we have to face the fact that the profound upheaval of the communication technology and the entire media landscape has completely changed our habitus of viewing the information environment and consuming news. There is little doubt that the deepening post-modernist culture will continue to advocate for interpretive flexibility and encourage every single individual to define the reality independently of any authoritative or monopolistic discourses – the future is bound to be an era where one can keep witnessing the "death of the author". Communication technologies will also continue to rush toward the directionality of decentralization, seeking to realize the complete activation of individual agency. Tech users, too, will celebrate their supposed realization of online democracy in one Internet frenzy after another, disregarding the costly civic responsibilities they have given up. Now that we seem powerless to reverse the directionality of the cultural and technological developments, our need for the systematic cultivation of news media literacy and critical news-consuming skills became stronger than ever before.

Index

Pages in *italics* refer to figures and pages in **bold** refer to tables.

For Product Safety Concerns and Information please contact our EU
representative GPSR@taylorandfrancis.com
Taylor & Francis Verlag GmbH, Kaufingerstraße 24, 80331 München, Germany

9 781032 625263